Stressful Life Events, Social-Support Networks, and Gerontological Health

Stressful Life Events, Social-Support Networks, and Gerontological Health

A Prospective Study

Thomas T.H. Wan
Virginia Commonwealth
University

LexingtonBooks
D.C. Heath and Company
Lexington, Massachusetts
Toronto

Library of Congress Cataloging in Publication Data

Wan, Thomas T.H.
  Stressful life events, social-support networks, and gerontological health.

  Bibliography: p.
  Includes index.
  1. Aged—United States. 2. Retirement—Psychological aspects.
3. Stress (Psychology) 4. Aged—Medical care—United States.
I. Title.
HQ1064.U5W33   306'.38   81–48393
ISBN 0–669–05359–7   AACR2

Published simultaneously in Canada

Printed in the United States of America

International Standard Book Number: 0–669–05359–7

Library of Congress Catalog Card Number: 81–48393

To Clara Chassell Cooper, Ph.D.,
a respected teacher and a scholar

Contents

List of Figures
and Tables

Acknowledgments

This work was supported by the National Institute on Aging under a research grant number 5-RO1-AGO1680-02.

I wish to acknowledge the contributions of my research associates, Barbara Gill Odell for chapters 4, 5, and 6, and Joyce Riley for chapter 8. They provided conceptual and technical expertise without which many of the chapters could not have been completed. I also would like to acknowledge my research assistants Wanda Mitchell and Li-Ching Hsu for preparing part of the annotated bibliography. In particular, I thank Mrs. Francine Meo for her patience and skillful typing of many versions of this manuscript.

Finally, I give my deepest appreciation to my wife, Sylvia, for her understanding, encouragement, and sacrifices. Without her support I would not have been able to embark upon this research project.

Introduction

The relationship between retirement and the well-being of older Americans is not clearly understood; retirement may have both positive and negative consequences. The withdrawal from an active work role in later life may mean a relief from a demanding and boring routine to some people, but it may also be a significant change that generates stress and requires the development of proper coping resources and the use of effective adaptive responses. In order to provide more systematic information for planning successful old age, it is imperative to examine empirically the issue of the effects of retirement on the physical and psychological status of the elderly. As Hamburg and Killilea [1] state, the medical-care system can more effectively serve its societal functions if the relationships among life stress, illness, patient behavior, and social-support systems are better understood. Furthermore, the study of short-term, as well as long-term, effects on health of role losses (including retirement and its concomitant changes in later life) may increase our understanding of aging as a complex social phenomenon.

This book presents findings from a panel study of the impact of major life changes occurring in later life on health status and health-care use. We assess the effect of retirement on health based on four waves (1969, 1971, 1973, and 1975) of panel data obtained from the Longitudinal Retirement History Study, a ten-year study of the retirement process conducted by the Social Security Administration. Furthermore, we determine the presumed effectiveness of social-support systems or social resources in minimizing any adverse impact of life transitions on the well-being of older people in the United States.

More specifically, the objectives of the research are

1. To develop a social-stress model viewing health-services utilization by the elderly in terms of responses to adverse effects of life-change events.
2. To identify components of life-change events in the retirement process in terms of major role loss.
3. To examine how life-change events and social-support systems independently affect utilization behavior.
4. To portray the sociodemographic and health characteristics of those who have experienced a variety of changes in later life.
5. To formulate a process of program intervention that will promote coping and preventive behavior in health maintenance in dealing with stress in later life.

Chapter 1 provides a theoretical overview of determinants of health of the elderly in terms of a social-stress model. Chapter 2 summarizes research methodology. Subsequent sections of this book present pertinent empirical findings on retirement and gerontological health in detail: chapter 3, validation of the concept of health and health-status change; chapter 4, role loss as a stressful event in later life; chapter 5, health effects of retirement; chapter 6, the role of social-support networks; chapter 7, gerontological health and social-support networks; and chapter 8, factors affecting health-services use. Finally, chapter 9 provides a synthesis of the research results and implications for retirement planning and outlines a preventive strategy for handling life stress in later life.

Reference

1. Hamburg, B.A., and M. Killilea, "Relation of Social Support, Stress, Illness, and Use of Health Services," *Healthy People,* the Surgeon General's Report on Health Promotion and Disease Prevention-Background Paper (Washington: Government Printing Office, 1979).

Stressful Life Events, Social-Support Networks, and Gerontological Health

1 Major Life Changes and Gerontological Health

The coincidence of two events in this century, the stabilization of modern industrialized economies and the unprecedented growth of the elderly population, has produced a unique social phenomenon: retirement. The leaving of employment with the intention of remaining unemployed, or retirement, may occur under a variety of circumstances. It may be voluntary (retirement for health reasons, or the decision to enjoy long-awaited leisure pursuits) or it may be forced (retirement because of mandatory age requirements).

Ill-defined as a social role, sometimes called the roleless role [1], retirement and the duties and obligations it entails have been probed most extensively in psychological research that looks at attitudes, life satisfaction, and activities in retirement. Sociological research has primarily confined itself to the issue of the centrality of the work role in the individual's life by studying whether retirement affects participation in other social roles such as the husband-wife relationship, friendship patterns, and community participation.

Little is known about the factors influencing adaptive processes in retirement, or the health consequences of retirement for the individual; yet the loss of work role may greatly affect the retiree's self-image and future activity. We recognize that retirement may cause some hardship, especially for the poor. Less than 60 percent of elderly on the lower end of the income scale, and about 20 percent of low-income minority elderly have savings to draw on in retirement [2]. In addition, circumstances relatively out of the individual's control, such as the rate of inflation, availability of Social Security and similar supplements, and access to community services, may also aggravate the problems of retirement. Still, we do not understand specifically what this impact is. Most research has considered retirement as a static state; yet some of those who retire eventually return to the labor force or continue to work part time. We must recognize that retirement need not be an either/or situation, but may be considered a gradual withdrawal from the labor market [3, 4]. Furthermore, retirement may occur concomitantly with other life events, such as widowhood, departure of mature children from home, change of living arrangement, and so forth. The determination of whether or not retirement and concomitant life events adversely affect health status of the elderly may improve our understanding of the social

1

etiology of life stress. In order to examine the dynamics of retirement and its health consequences, longitudinal research to follow a panel of the elderly is required.

Socially Induced Stress and Decline in Health: A Theoretical Perspective

Several theoretical models have attempted to define the biochemical, physiological, psychological, and sociocultural effects of stress [5–9]. In these models, stress generally has been defined as the "discomforting responses of persons in particular situations," [5] and as a "state manifested by a specific syndrome which consists of all the nonspecifically induced changes within the biologic syndrome." [8]

Models of stress also vary in their focus. While Mechanic [5] emphasizes coping behavior, Wolff [7] looks at bodily adjustment to stress-producing stimuli; Seyle, [8] with his general adaptation syndrome, proposes a biochemical model of stress that consists of the following three steps: (1) an alarm reaction, (2) a stage of resistance, and, finally, (3) a stage of exhaustion if the stress continues. On the other hand, Dohrenwend and Dohrenwend [9] focus on the role of support in mediating the effects of stress.

Previous models of reactions to stress have been criticized for their failure to agree on a universal definition of stress, and for their specificity in limiting the study of the effects of stress to biochemical, physiological, psychological, or sociocultural reactions. What is needed, according to Scott and Howard [10], is a more comprehensive theory of the effects of stress. Our study examines the effects of a particular stressful experience, retirement, on several dimensions of health.

In the past decade, a great deal of research in medical sociology has focused on the sociopathogenesis of mental and physical illness. One of the factors studied has been social stress induced by life-change events. It is generally assumed that the greater life change an individual experiences, the more he must adapt. Maladaption or an inadequate coping process may disturb bodily functions, making an individual more susceptible to illness. Recently, the role of the social network—family, peers, and the community—has been pursued as a factor in determining ability to cope with life change.

While many empirical studies have been generated by the foregoing assumptions, little research has dealt specifically with the effect of life-change events on the elderly's illness level and illness behavior; yet this group experiences life changes of considerable magnitude (as widowhood, retirement, and change of residence). This group also has an increasing need for health services. Although health status, specifically chronicity of illness, accounts for much of the variation in health-services utilization, it is possible that life-change events precipitate the decline in physical and mental well-being and induce utilization of services. It is also likely that the social network mediates such a pattern. These findings could have relevance for the development of preventive measures such as psychological counseling, friendly visiting, and, possibly, financial subsidies to families to strengthen weak networks, as forms of primary prevention.

Life-Change Events and Onset of Illness

Life change, as a multidimensional concept, includes the extent of change in a specific period as well as qualities such as desirability and preferability. The change may occur in many different spheres, that is, financial, occupational, marital, interpersonal, and residential.

Several studies have documented the relationship between stress, as measured by the number and magnitude of life events, and health status. The Schedule of Recent Experience (SRE) of Holmes and Rahe [11], which lists forty-three life-change events, is the most frequently employed measure of change. Each SRE item is quantified by a certain number of life change units (LCU's), ranging from 11 to 100. The scale was derived by arbitrarily assigning a weight of 50 to the marriage event and by using samples of convenience to assign rates of 1 to 100 to all other events, with marriage as the reference value. A one-to-two-year span (prior to the administration of the scale) has become the conventional perspective for life-change measurement. Scores of 150 to 199 LCUs have been identified as a mild life crisis; 200–299 LCUs as a moderate life crisis; and 300 LCUs or more as a major life crisis.

Rahe et al. [12] report on the relationship between life change and health using military records for a sample of servicemen who were discharged in 1958 because of psychiatric illness diagnosed while on active duty. Information on both illness experience and life change was collected from service records, and psychiatric social histories. These patterns were examined for each year of active duty. Both variables tended to cluster in certain years, and cluster years of life change were generally seen to occur immediately prior to an illness or illness cluster. Further, there was a significant difference between the degree of life change and the severity of the succeeding illness. Within the sample of individual case histories presented here, there were two instances of death for individuals with high life-change scores. The sample was, of course, deliberately selected to include persons who were ill (discharged for disability) in order to investigate the temporal relationship beteen life change and illness.

Pesznecker and McNeil [3] utilized the SRE scale along with other measures to investigate factors that might intervene to enable individuals in the general population to withstand a high degree of life change. These other measures were health habits (a nineteen-item questionnaire constructed by the authors to address health practices accepted by professionals as useful to health maintenance); alterations in health status (a yes or no response to a major change in health during the past two years); psychological well-being (an eight-item, single-score index developed by Bradburn and Caplovitz [14]), and social assets past and present (based on a scale developed by Luborsky [15]). Data were analyzed from 548 mail questionnaires completed by a systematic sample of residents of Renton, Washington. The authors' hypothesis that health habits, psychological well-being, and social assets might temper health changes associated with life changes was not supported. The strongest relationship was the positive association between life change and health status.

Although the other variables investigated evidenced only a weak association with major health change, all were in the expected direction (for example, psychological well-being was inversely related to reported major health change). When LCE scores were dichotimized above and below the sample mean, there was no correlation between LCE level and major health change. Sex was significantly correlated with major health change, but women tended to report more major health change compared to men, regardless of LCE score. Social class also had a significant effect on the relationship between LCE score and major health change: correlations were much higher for high than for low social-class respondents. The authors indicate that a prospective study may be necessary to understand why one group is able to avoid illness in the face of high life change.

Wyler [16] found that the magnitude of life events was positively related to the seriousness of illness among those with chronic, but not with acute, illnesses. In a prospective study covering a two-year period, Myers et al. [17] also documented an increase in mental illness among those with an increase in life-change events. Furthermore, classifying the majority of studies on stressful life events, they found that the "relocation event," which involved moving, did not affect the occurrence of mental illness, while events classified as changes in social field, involving the exit—but not the entrance—of an individual, did. Stein and Susser [18] also discovered an increase in mental illness following bereavement.

Other variables, such as class and previous experience with stress, have been shown to confound the relationship between stress and health status [19, 20]. While previous studies have not dealt specifically with the aged, it is possible to glean indications of the relationship of changes to health and health-care use.

Retirement and Its Health Consequences

The retirement process, which is so often the portal through which the adaptation for role loss starts, can easily become the precipitating agent for mental and physical disorders. According to life-stress theory, retirement may be considered a stress-inducing factor that may have an adverse effect on health in the elderly. This statement remains speculative if no systematic research, using prospective-study designs, validates this assumption.

In studying a large sample of noninstitutionalized men and women aged sixty-five and older, Thompson [21] indicated that most of the variation in morale between the retired and the employed was explained by four variables: perception of health, age, income, and functional disability. When these factors were controlled, there was very little difference between the working and the retired men who perceived themselves in poorer health, had more functional disability, or had lower incomes because they were older and not simply because they were retired. Similarly, Mutran and Reitzes [22], basing their information on a survey of 4,254 elders conducted by the National Council on Aging in 1974, reported that, everything being equal, retired men are not significantly different from working men in assessing their subjective well-being. They found that well-being of the elderly was not directly related to retirement, but that it was directly related to the extent of community activities in which individuals were involved. These findings support the fact that changes in psychological health cannot be directly attributed to retirement itself [23].

A study by Jacobson [24] of preretirement semi-skilled workers found that women are less inclined to be retirement-oriented than men and are more likely to propose older "ideal" ages for retirement. They attach greater value to work-based social ties, and view work as a guarantee against loneliness. This concurs with Streib and Schneider's findings, which showed women felt more useless than men at the time of retirement [23]. Both of these studies indicate that retirement may be a more stressful experience for women than for men. With more women choosing careers outside the home, this could be a significant factor for future cohorts of women.

In a study of male semi-skilled workers, Glamser [25] found that the worker's attitude toward retirement appears to be more influenced by the individual's total situation than by the loss of worker role. Therefore, workers who can realistically expect a positive retirement experience are more likely to have a positive attitude toward retirement. According to this study, the loss of work role in itself does not appear to be devastating to health. Glamser and DeJong [26] found that group discussions, as a form of preretirement counseling, were effective in reducing uncertainty about the future and in increasing the worker's feeling of preparedness for retirement.

Although some clinical case examples suggest that the impact of retirement may be traumatic, research studies, [27, 28] for the most part, do not support this. Instead, most research concludes that retirement may lead to lowered morale in the elderly, but that lowered morale does not automatically occur with retirement [23]. The emotional impact of retirement is based on the cumulative effect of all those factors that affect individuals regardless of age—such as socioeconomic status, personality, health status, marital status, range of interests, vigor, and attitudes toward work.

To summarize, previous research seems to indicate that retirement as a life-change event is not as stressful as expected. Women appear to be more negatively affected by retirement than are men. Conditions surrounding retirement, such as state of health and level of income, may be as important in determining morale and attitude after retirement as the actual loss of work role. In the present research, we are interested in investigating the role loss resulting from retirement and its cumulative effects, with other life events, on health and use of health services.

Life Stress and Coping Resources

In reviewing the current literature, we found that (1) stress may affect the perception and interpretation of symptoms, and (2) that stress may also affect the decision to seek care or to adopt a sick role. For example, in a study of physician utilization, Roghmann and Haggerty [29] reported that, when no illness was present, stress tended to increase the probability of health-service utilization; however, stress increased utilization of only certain types of contacts, that is, telephone calls, and visits to the emergency departments and outpatient departments rather than to private-physician offices where the appointment system created a barrier. These findings corroborated those of Greenley and Mechanic [30], who found that the magnitude of stress was related not only to whether help was sought for psychological problems, but also to the source of care chosen.

Social support can be defined as support accessible to an individual through social ties to other individuals, groups, and the larger community [31]. These social ties represent a support system that may provide not only emotional (expressive) support, but also instrumental support, including goods, services, monetary aids, and so on. Social support is seen as a mediating force that helps the individual cope with, or adapt to, stress or a life crisis. It is also considered one of the coping or adaptive resources that serves to prevent, avoid, or control emotional distress [32].

Mechanic [33] describes three components of successful personal adaptation: (1) the individual must have coping abilities or the capabilities and skills to deal with social and environmental demands; (2) he or she must have motivation to meet demands; and (3) he or she must be capable of maintaining a state of psychological equilibrium, so energies and skills can be directed to meeting external, in contrast to internal, needs. He further states that the ability of individuals to maintain psychological comfort will depend, not only on their intrapsychic resources, but also on the social supports available in their environment [33].

Several empirical studies consider social-support systems as buffering factors between stressful life events and illness [34, 35, 17]. In studying the experience of involuntary job loss of the aged, Gore [35] compared two groups of recently unemployed males, one with low and the other with high social support. She found that, while no differences existed in reemployment rates or the amount of economic deprivation experienced, the group with higher social support manifested less self-blame and depression and had fewer physiological symptoms of illness. Her findings pertain to the situation of the involuntarily retired male and suggest the buffering effect of support. The value of support for the elderly in mitigating other changes involving loss is also documented. Lowenthal and Haven [36] report that, among their elderly sample, those who decreased their social interaction and who did not have confidantes were more often depressed than those with confidantes or increased interaction. In the area of bereavement, Cobb [37] reviewed several empirical studies and reported that there was an inverse relationship between contact with others and risk of mental illness.

The utilization literature consistently points to the positive association between physical functioning and use of health services [38, 39, 40]. However, the cause-effect relationship between health and use of health services cannot be ascertained by the analysis of data collected from a cross-sectional survey. In order to study the effects on the use of health services of various concomitants of life change in the retirement process, we need to examine data collected from a longitudinal panel study.

Analytical Models

Many models of utilization behavior have been developed in the health-services research field. These include economic models [41, 42] and social- or behavioral-systems models [43, 44, 45, 46]. One frequently used model, employing three basic determinants of utilization behavior as a theoretical framework, was developed by Andersen [43] in his study of differences in family use of health services. The first dimension is predisposing factors that exist prior to the onset of illness. These are used as predictor variables of the propensity to seek care. The second dimension is enabling conditions that may facilitate or impede use of services. The third dimension pertains to illness level, either perceived illness or symptoms evaluated by the professional.

In our research, the major interest is in assessing the relative effects of concomitant life-change events in the retirement process on the use of health services. Our analytical framework is based upon a revised version of Andersen's behavioral model [43], which will help to classify various life-change events in later life into the three basic dimensions noted above (see figure 1-1).

Implications of the differences between cross-sectional and longitudinal data have not yet been fully incorporated into health-services research on aging. In previous research, for instance, the possibility of confounding

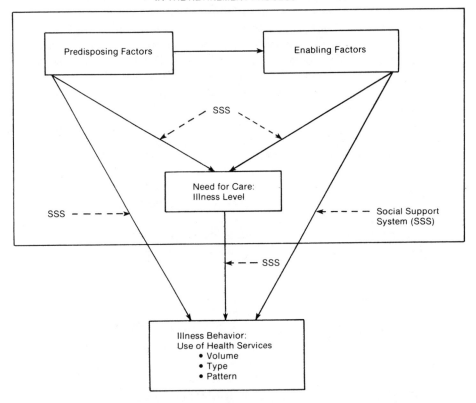

CONCOMITANT LIFE CHANGE EVENTS
IN THE RETIREMENT PROCESS

Figure 1-1. Theoretical Model of Effects of Life-Change Events and Social Support on Use of Health Services

effects of social support and role change on need for care has not been addressed. Furthermore, our study will examine whether or not the debilitating experience of role changes, either positive or negative, is what causes the increase in need for care among the elderly. The use of panel data, which allows us to measure the level of health status before observing any change in need for care over time, can delineate the causal relationship between life-change events, social support, and use of health services.

In analyzing the effects of life-change events and social support, we have further specified three submodels in terms of retirement status. The first model will examine the net effect of life-change events subsequent to retirement on health status and use of health services (see model 1). This approach will compare retirees to nonretirees and follow them up for a period so that life-change events resulting from retirement can be determined.

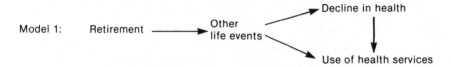

The second model will examine the synergistic effects of retirement and other life-change events on health status and use of health services; retirement is considered as a concomitant of other life-change events. This approach can investigate the relative influence of retirement and other life-change events on use of health services.

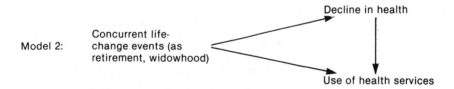

The third model will examine the role of social support on mediating the effects of stressful life events resulting from role losses on health status and health-care use.

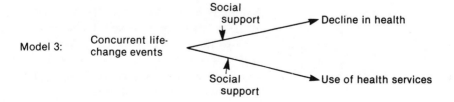

A review of existing research [46–50], shows a possible link between life-change events, social support, health status, and service utilization. The discovery of a causal link for the elderly among these variables could have relevance of future policy on aging. In addition, such findings may enhance understanding of the phenomenon of stress in later life. For example, if retirement affects health and health care, it will have profound policy implications for the development of health and rehabilitation programs for the elderly. On the national level, the magnitude of the need for care among the preretirement population should be identified and estimated by carefully executed research. In answering the general question, what are the effects of retirement on health and health care, two approaches can be taken. We can simply study whether or not older adults use more health services as a result of changes in the need for care or in illness level in the process of retirement; or we can study the concomitant effects of retirement and other related factors, such as decline of health status, on health care of the elderly. However, there remain many unanswered questions. This research is an attempt to answer the following questions: (1) Does the increase of health services utilization occur as a result of retirement? (2) Do changes in life events (including income, living arrangements, and so forth) during the retirement process affect the use of health services, when changes in illness levels are controlled? (3) Does the increase of the use of health services result from the decline of physical functions after retirement? (4) What are the characteristics of retirees versus nonretirees in the elderly population, those who will most likely use health services?

Three testable hypotheses are formulated in terms of the three models stated in the former section:

Hypothesis 1:   The larger the degree of life-change events occurring subsequent to retirement, the greater the decline in health status among the retirees; consequently, retirees will use more health services than nonretirees.

Hypothesis 2:   Retirement and its concomitant changes in the process of retirement are directly related to the decline in health status and use of health services.

Hypothesis 3:   Among older adults, the larger the degree of life-change events evoked, the more frequently they will experience a decline in health status; however, this relationship will be substantially reduced if a strong social-support network is present.

Summary

In this chapter we have set forth a social-stress framework designed to ensure that the decline in health and increase in use of health services will be accounted for by the study of role losses and other significant life-change events in later life. We believe that this conceptual framework can facilitate our interpretation of findings from the analysis of Longitudinal Retirement History Study (LRHS). In the next chapter we begin to provide the detailed description of LRHS data and analytical methods used in this book.

References

1. Shanas, Ethel, "Adjustment to Retirement: Substitution or Accommodation" in Francis M. Carp, ed., *Retirement,* (New York: Behavioral Publications, 1972).

2. Harris, L. and Associates. *Myth and Reality of Aging in America,* (Washington, D.C.: National Council of Aging, 1975).

3. Carp, F.M. *The Retirement Process* (Washington, D.C.: U.S. Department of Health, Education and Welfare, 1968).

4. Hendricks, J., and O. Hendricks, *Aging in Mass Society,* (Cambridge, Mass.: Winthrop Publishers, Inc., 1977).

5. Mechanic, D. *Students Under Stress* (New York: New York Free Press, 1962).

6. Basowitz, H., et al., *Anxiety and Stress* (New York: McGraw Hill, 1955).

7. Wolff, H.G., et al., *Life Stress and Bodily Disease,* (Baltimore, Md.: The Williams and Wilkins Co., 1950).

8. Seyle, H., *The Stress of Life* (New York: McGraw-Hill, 1956).

9. Dohrenwend, B.S., and B.P. Dohrenwend *Stress Life Events: Their Nature and Effects* (New York: Wiley and Sons, 1974).

10. Scott, R., and A. Howard, "Models of Stress" in S. Levine and N.A. Scotch, eds., *Social Stress* (Chicago, Ill.: Aldine Publishing Co., 1970).

11. Holmes, T.H., and R. Rahe, "The Social Readjustment Rating Scale," *Journal of Psychosomatic Research* 11 (1967):213-218.

12. Rahe, R.H., et al., "A Longitudinal Study of Life Change and Illness Patterns," *Journal of Psychosomatic Research* 10 (May 1967): 355-366.

13. Pesznecker, B.L., and J. McNeil, "Relationship Among Health Habits, Social Assets, Psychological Well-Being, Life Change, and Alterations in Health Status," *Nursing Research* 24 (1975):442-447.

14. Bradburn, N.M., and D. Caplovitz, *Reports on Happiness: A Pilot*

Study of Behavior Related to Mental Health. (Chicago, Ill.: Aldine Publishing Co., 1965).

15. Luborsky, L., et al., "A Self-Administered Social Assets Scale for Predicting Physical and Psychological Illness and Health," *Journal of Psychosomatic Research* 17 (1973):109–120.

16. Wyler, A., M. Masuda, and T.H. Holmes, "Magnitude of Life Events and Seriousness of Illness," *Psychosomatic Medicine* 33 (1971): 115–120.

17. Myers, J., J. Lindenthal, and M.P. Pepper, "Like Events and Mental Status: A Longitudinal Study," *Journal of Health and Social Behavior* 13 (1972):398–405.

18. Stein, Z., and M. Susser, "Widowhood and Mental Illness," *British Journal of Preventive and Social Medicine* 23 (1969):106–110.

19. Dohrenwend, B., "Psychiatric Disorder in General Populations: Problem of the Untreated Case," *American Journal of Public Health* 60 (June 1970):1052–1064.

20. Eaton, W.W., "Life Events, Social Supports, and Psychiatric Symptoms: A Reanalysis of New Haven Data," *Journal of Health and Social Behavior* 19 (1978):230–237.

21. Thompson, T.B., "Work Versus Leisure Roles: An Investigation of Morale Among Employed and Retired Men," *Journal of Gerontology* 28 (1973):339–344.

22. Mutran, E., and D.C. Reitzes, "Retirement, Identity and Well-Being: Realignment of Role Relationships," *Journal of Gerontology* 36, no. 6 (1981):733–740.

24. Streib, G., and G. Schneider, *Retirement in American Society* (Ithaca, New York: Cornell University Press, 1971).

24. Jacobson, D., "Rejection of the Retired Role: A Study of Female Industrial Workers in Their Future," *Human Relations* 27 (1974):477–492.

25. Glamser, F.D., "Determinants of a Positive Attitude Toward Retirement," *Journal of Gerontology* 30 (1976):595–600.

26. Glamser, F.D., and G.F. Dejong, "The Efficacy of Pre-Retirement Preparation Programs for Industrial Workers," *Journal of Gerontology* 30 (1975):395–600.

27. Holtzman, J.M., et al., "Health and Early Retirement Decisions," *Journal of the American Geriatric Society* 28 (1980):23–28.

28. Crawford, M.P., "Retirement as Psychosocial Crisis," *Journal of Psychosomatic Research* 16 (1972):375–380.

29. Roghmann, K.J., and R.J. Haggerty, "Family Stress and the Use of Health Services," *International Journal of Epidemiology* 1 (1972): 279–286.

30. Greenley, J., and D. Mechanic, "Patterns of Seeking Care for Psychological Problems," in D. Mechanic, *The Growth of Bureaucratic Medicine* (New York: John Wiley and Sons, 1976).

31. Lin, R., et al., "Social Support, Stressful Life Events and Illness: A Model and an Empirical Test." *Journal of Health and Social Behavior* 20 (1979):108–120.

32. Pearlin, L.I., and C. Shooler, "The Structure of Coping," *Journal of Health and Social Behavior* 19 (1978):2–21.

33. Mechanic, D., "Social Structure and Personal Adaptation: Some Neglected Dimensions," in G.V. Coehlo, D.A. Hamburg, and J.E. Adams, eds., *Coping and Adaptation,* (New York: Basic Books, 1974).

34. Caplan, Gerald, *Support Systems and Community Mental Health: Lectures on Concept Development* (New York: Behavioral Publications, 1974).

35. Gore, S., "The Effects of Social Support in Moderating the Health Consequences of Unemployment," *Journal of Health and Social Behavior* 19 (1978):157–165.

36. Lowenthal, M.F., and C. Haven, "Interaction and Adaptation: Intimacy as Critical Variable," *American Sociological Review* 33 (1968): 20–30.

37. Cobb, S., "Social Support as Moderator of Life Stress," *Psychosomatic Medicine* 38 (1976):300–314.

38. Wan, T.T.H., and B.G. Odell, "Factors Affecting the Use of Social and Health Services Among the Elderly," *Aging and Society* 1, no. 1 (March 1981):95–118.

39. Davis, D., and R. Reynolds, "Medicare and the Utilization of Health Care Services by the Elderly," *Journal of Human Resources* 10 (1975):361–377.

40. German, P.S., E.A. Skinner and S. Shapiro, "Ambulatory Care for Chronic Conditions in an Inner City Elderly Population," *American Journal of Public Health* 66 (1976):660–666.

41. Feldstein, Paul J., "Research on the Demand for Health Services," *Milbank Memorial Fund Quarterly* 44 (July 1966):128–162.

42. Wirick, G., "A Multiple Equation Model of Demand for Health Care," *Health Services Research* 1 (1966):301–346.

43. Andersen, R., "A Behavioral Model of Families' Use of Services." *Research Series #25.* (Chicago Ill.: Center for Health Administration Studies, 1968).

44. Andersen, R., and J. Newman, "Societal and Individual Determinants of Medical Care Utilization in the United States," *Milbank Memorial Fund Quarterly* 51 (1973):95–124.

45. Wan, T.H., and S. Soifer, "Determinants of Physician Utilization: A Causal Analysis," *Journal of Health and Social Behavior* 15 (1974): 100–108.

46. Haynes, S.G., et al., "The Relationship of Normal Involuntary Retirement to Early Mortality Among U.S. Rubber Workers," *Social Science and Medicine* 11 (1977):105–114.

47. Kaitaranta, H., and T. Purola, "A Systems-Oriented Approach to the Consumption of Medical Commodities," *Social Science and Medicine* 7 (1973):531–540.

48. Stokes, R.G., and G.L. Maddox, "Some Social Factors in Retirement Adaptation," *Journal of Gerontology* 22 (1967):329–333.

49. Mutran, E., and D.C. Reitzes, "Retirement, Identity and Well-Being: Realignment of Role Relationships," *Journal of Gerontology* 36, no. 6 (1981):733–740.

50. Martin, J., and A. Doran, "Evidence Concerning the Relationship Between Health and Retirement," *Sociological Review* 14 (1966):329.

51. Minkler, M., "Research on the Health Effects of Retirement: An Uncertain Legacy," *Journal of Health and Social Behavior* 13 (1981): 398–405.

2 The Study Sample and Analytical Methods

In the review of the literature on life-change-events research, many criticisms of methodological problems in employing a cross-sectional-study design have been noted [1-3]. For instance, the causal relationship between life events and illness cannot be ascertained since the temporal sequence of change events collected from retrospective studies cannot be precisely determined. Furthermore, the recall of events may be affected by selective memory bias; thus the reliability of self-reported life experiences is questionable.

In order to determine whether or not life-change events have played either a direct or an indirect role in affecting health and health-care use, we employed a prospective study design in which a panel group was selected and information was obtained to determine if different kinds of life events resulting from role losses, such as retirement, widowhood, and departure of mature children from home, impacts on the variation in illness and illness behavior of older adults. Moreover, the follow-up study of health of a selected sample population in the years after retirement can clearly reveal the causal chain between retirement and health.

Study Design

Source of Data

The data for this research are based on the Longitudinal Retirement History Study (LRHS) conducted by the Social Security Administration to study the retirement attitudes, plans, resources, and activities of older Americans [4]. The original sample of the 1969 LRHS consisted of 11,153 noninstitutionalized civilians, aged fifty-eight to sixty-three, who were either (1) married and unmarried men, or (2) unmarried women. These individuals constituted a sample drawn by stratified random-cluster sampling procedures as used in the Current Population Survey of the Bureau of the Census. The respondents were revisited every other year during a period of ten years (1969-1979). The interview schedule consisted of six major parts: labor-force history; retirement and retirement plans; health and health care; household, family, and social activities; income, assets, and debts; and

spouse's labor-force history. The follow-up survey of 1971 interviewed
9,924 people previously studied in 1969, plus 245 surviving spouses. By
1973, the second follow-up survey reinterviewed 8,928 individuals. Of 2,225
who were not reinterviewed, 984 were deaths and the remainder either
refused to participate or could not be located. Of the 8,716 interviewed in
1975, 727 were surviving spouses of original respondents.

Description of Study Sample

A considerable amount of evidence has shown that poor health causes early
retirement, yet the adverse effect of retirement on health, and its concomitant life-change events have not been thoroughly substantiated in previous
studies. The present research has adopted a prospective study design:
respondents to LRHS who were working and had no functional limitations
in 1969 are included in the panel study. This restriction identified a total of
5,884 people, about 54 percent of the LRHS sample for our prospective
study (table 2-1). There were more married males, urban residents, and
white-collar workers in the prospective study sample than in the other subgroups. Detailed information on the study sample is presented in tables 2-2
and 2-3.

Table 2-1
Retirement and Disability Status of 10,905 Respondents in the 1969
Retirement-History Study, by Selected Characteristics
(percentage)

| | Retirement Status in 1969 | | | |
| | Retired | | Working | |
Characteristics	Disabled	Not Disabled	Disabled	Not Disabled
Total percentage	17.6	7.4	21.0	54.0
	(1,920)	(807)	(2,294)	(5,884)
White	83.1	93.3	89.6	90.9
Males	72.0	54.9	77.9	76.7
Married males	80.2	83.5	87.5	89.4
Urban	62.0	69.6	65.0	73.1
Completed high school	9.9	21.3	14.0	20.4
White-collar workers	5.0	12.1	19.2	31.0
Service workers	88.8	80.0	56.1	41.2

Note: Of the original sample, respondents who had never worked and who reported no occupation were excluded from this table.

Table 2-2
The Prospective Study Sample, by Selected Social and Demographic Characteristics, in 1969

Characteristics	Number	Percentage
Age		
58 years	1,280	21.8
59 years	1,061	18.0
60 years	1,019	17.3
61 years	952	16.2
62 years	880	15.0
63 years	687	11.7
Educational attainment		
Under 9th grade	2,024	34.3
Some high school	2,662	45.2
High school graduate/college education	1,198	20.4
Occupational group		
White-collar workers	1,823	31.0
Blue-collar workers	1,373	23.3
Service workers	2,423	41.2
Farm managers and workers	212	3.6
Unknown	53	0.9
Residential background		
Urban	4,303	73.1
Rural	1,581	26.9

$N = 5,884$

Note: When persons did not report current occupations, their previous occupations were used.

Table 2-3
Characteristics of the Prospective Study Sample, by Survey Year

| Characteristics | Survey Year | | | |
	1969	1971	1973	1975
Total (100 percent)	5,884	5,386	5,107	4,748
Marital status/sex				
Married men	68.6	67.1	64.2	59.1
Nonmarried men	8.1	9.6	12.4	18.0
Married women	0.0	0.8	1.1	2.9
Nonmarried women	23.2	22.5	22.3	20.0
Retirement status				
Retired	0.0	23.9	53.3	75.0
Working	100.0	76.1	46.7	25.0
Disability status				
Disabled	0.0			
Not disabled	100.0			

The study sample includes those who were not retired and had no functional disabilities reported in 1969.

In the study sample, approximately 40 percent were under sixty years of age, 20.4 percent were high school graduates or had a college education, 31 percent had a white-collar occupation, and 73.1 percent had an urban residential background (table 2-2). To aid in comparing changes in retirement and disability conditions, table 2-3 provides an overview of respondents in each of the four years of the LRHS—1969, 1971, 1973, and 1975. In the six years during which the study sample aged from 58–63 to 64–69, a substantial increase (from 8.1 percent to 18.0 percent) occurred in the proportion of nonmarried men, while there was a slight decline in nonmarried women (from 23.2 percent to 20.0 percent). As would be expected, there was a steady increase in the proportion considering themselves retired, a biannual rate of 25 percent. By 1975, only one-third of the study sample were still working. As expected, there was a decline in physical health as the study population aged; about one-third of them had functional limitations by 1975.

Analytical Methods

Basing our investigation on four waves (1969, 1971, 1973, and 1975) of panel data obtained from the Retirement History Study, we carried out the following analysis, using multivariate approaches.

Multiple-Indicators Approach

In examining the stability of measures of health over time, we formulated a three-wave, one-indicator model for each of the three health indicators (self-assessed health, life satisfaction, and disability). The reliability and stability coefficients are estimated with the use of a panel-study design [5]. The specification of statistical models are presented in the appropriate sections in chapter 3.

Multiple-Classification Analysis

In order to provide relevant policy recommendations, we used multiple-classification analysis (MCA) to identify social, demographic, and other-related profiles of the older adults who were most likely to have poorer health status and use more health services.

MCA is used to examine the effects of the variables in explaining total physician visits and hospitalization. This analytical technique examines the interrelationships between several predictors and a dependent variable within the context of an additive model [6]. MCA is similar to dummy-variable regression, the major exception being that coefficients for each category of the predictor are expressed as deviations from the grand mean of the dependent variable, while in dummy-variable regression they are expressed in terms of the deviation of the one category of the predictor from the omitted (reference) category. MCA shares the advantage of dummy-variable regression in that the relationships among the variables need not be linear.

Path Analysis

In analyzing panel data, we have a great opportunity to formulate a social-stress model, using health status and physician utilization as endogeneous (dependent) variables, and life events and social-support networks as exogeneous variables. According to conventional path analysis, the correlation coefficient may be considered as the total independent effect of an independent variable on a dependent variable. The total effect consists of the direct causal effect (beta or path coefficient), indirect causal effect, and association due to intercorrelation between the independent variable and predetermined variables. The indirect causal effect measures the effect of a variable through the various paths linking it to a dependent variable [7–9].

In addition to multivariate analyses, we performed descriptive statistical analyses, providing the social and demographic profiles of those who had experienced such role losses as retirement, widowhood, and so forth.

References

1. Rabkin, J.G., and E.L. Struening, "Life Events, Stress and Illness," *Science* 194 (1976):1013–1020.

2. Gore, S., "Stress-Buffering Functions of Social Supports: An Appraisal and Clarification of Research Models," in B.S. Dohrenwend and B.P. Dohrenwend, eds., *Life Stress and Illness* (New York: Neale Watson, 1981).

3. Eckenrode, J., and S. Gore, "Stressful Events and Social Supports: The Significance of Context," in B.H. Gottlieb ed., *Social Networks and Social Support in Community Mental Health* (Beverly Hills., Cal.: Sage Publications, Inc., 1981).

4. Irelan, L.M., "Retirement History Study: Introduction" "Retirement History Study Report No. 1," *Social Security Bulletin.* (Washington, D.C.: Dept. HEW-Social Security Administration, 1972).

5. Sullivan, J.L., and S. Feldman, *Multiple Indicators: An Introduction* (Beverly Hills, Cal.: Sage Publications, 1979).

6. Andrews, F.M., J.N. Morgan, and J.A. Sonquist, *Multiple Classification Analysis* (Ann Arbor, Michigan. Survey Research Center, Institute for Social Research, The University of Michigan, 1969).

7. Anderson, J., "Demographic Factors Affecting Health Services Utilization: A Causal Model," *Medical Care* 11 (March–April 1973): 104–120.

8. Finney, J.M., "Indirect Effects in Path Analysis," *Sociological Methods and Research* 1 (1972):175–186.

9. Wan, Thomas T.H., and S. Soifer, "Determinants of Physician Utilization: A Causal Analysis," *Journal of Health and Social Behavior* 15 (1974):100–108.

3 Validating the Construct of Health

There has been considerable interest in the formulation of an index of personal-health status for a general population, one based on subjective assessments [1–6] and objective measures [7–9]. Several recent studies have provided some evidence of the validity and reliability of the measures-of-health-status as important indicators of the quality of life [10–12]. However, none of these studies has systematically examined the stability of the health index over time. In the past, multiple measures of the construct of health have been made at roughly the same time in cross-sectional study designs.

In evaluating the health index, the following suggested criteria should be considered:

1. Precision of the measure: to obtain reliable data.
2. Relevance of the measure: to measure what it purports to measure.
3. Predictability of the measure: to construct a health-status index based on known factors affecting the health or well-being of the population; to be able to use it to predict the actual state of health.
4. Applicability of the measure: to ascertain the availability of data at a reasonable cost; to identify the differences in various states of health; to discriminate between the true states of good health and poor health; to define the comparability of indicators used; to interpret the results with consideration of population variation.
5. Stability of the measure: to determine the correlations between the measure at two time points or waves.

The first evaluative criterion, precision, refers to the reliability of the measure. A test-retest procedure can be applied to compute a reliability coefficient. Sometimes, the repeated measuring of the same items in a selected subsample can produce an estimate of reliability, that is, correlation coefficient. Relevance, the second criterion, is concerned with validity and deals with the substance of the measure: content validity, construct validity, and predictive validity [13, 14]. A detailed and systematic analysis of validity can be found in recent methodological literature [15–17].

The third criterion, predictability, is related to the total variance in

21

health status explained by pertinent health indicators in the confirmatory multivariate analysis [18]. The fourth criterion, applicability of the measure, is a complex one that deserves more attention in the health field. According to epidemiological research, two simple tests of applicability can be used: sensitivity and specificity. Sensitivity is the capacity to predict poor health in those who perceive themselves in poor health. Specificity is the capacity to identify those in good health when they actually perceive themselves in good health.

The last criterion is the stability of health measure over time. The correlation between the unobserved variable over time is an estimate of stability of the (observed) health indicator.

These criteria are not mutually exclusive, so that one may be stressed more than another by the researcher. Current research on health status has been concentrated on the evaluation of reliability (criterion 1) and validity (criterion 2) of the scales developed [19, 20, 21].

There has been virtually no systematic work evaluating health status indexes by focusing on all five evaluative criteria as suggested.

This chapter describes an attempt using a multiple indicators approach to examine the reliability and stability of health measures in terms of subjectively assessed health, life satisfaction, and physical disability in a panel-study design. Furthermore, the adequacy of these health indicators will be validated by a multivariate analysis, using health indicators as predictor variables of health-care behavior, that is, use of health services.

Related Research

Although there have been diverse approaches to studying the level of well-being, the identification of components of health has received relatively little attention. Most gerontological studies of personal health status focus on issues dealing with the relationship of age to subjectively assessed health and life satisfaction.

Aging and Health

In a recent work, Shanas and Maddox [22] gave a comprehensive overview of research findings on aging and health. In discussing patterns of morbidity, they remarked on the commonly observed association between illness and socioeconomic level and contended that the higher prevalence of disease among lower socioeconomic groups is attributable to differences in life-style and access to health care. The greater morbidity, but lower mortality, rate for females was also noted. In reviewing the studies, they found that whites enjoy better health than nonwhites in that they have fewer restricted activity days and less disability. Shanas and Maddox also cited the increase in the prevalence of chronic disease with age, along with dental, visual, and hearing problems. These authors maintained that illness and disability have a negative effect on self-esteem and sense of well-being, and they related physical illness to mental illness in the older age groups.

Shanas [23] noted two major approaches to health status and health-needs assessment among the elderly: the medical model, which stresses the importance of physical examination, and the functional model, which relies on self-assessments of health and functional status. Differing interpretations of health resulting from application of these two models reflect the fact that the medical model is based on absolute levels of health rather than on levels relative to age and sex. Maddox and Douglass [24] used an approach that combined the two models. They made a longitudinal comparison of physician and patient health ratings and found that ratings tend to be congruent over time and that the individual's rating was the more reliable predictor of future physician's rating. This finding lends support to the use of subjective measures as reliable data.

Kovar [25], investigating the health status of the elderly, wrote that two-thirds of the noninstitutionalized elderly report that their health is good or excellent, while 9 percent report that their health is poor compared to others their age. The nonwhite elderly report poor health twice as often as do the white elderly. Kovar also made the important observation that health status among persons in the same age group varies greatly, but that, on the average, people in their 60s and early 70s are in far better health than those in older age groups.

The danger of broad generalization in research dealing with aging is well illustrated in a study by Spreitzer and Snyder [26] in which they found that women report a higher degree of life satisfaction than men from age eighteen through age sixty-five, at which time life satisfaction increases for men and decreases for women. Although their study is cross-sectional, similar findings have been reported in longitudinal studies by Palmore [27] and Streib and Schneider [28].

In terms of health status, differences between the sexes have most often shown females to have higher rates of morbidity, while males have higher mortality rates. In fact, it has been a long-standing observation that "women are sicker, but men die sooner." Verbrugge [29] suggested that interview and illness behavior related to social and psychological factors tend to inflate female morbidity rates. Nathanson [30] advanced the supposition that observed sex differences in morbidity may also be influenced by physician behavior. Larson [31], however, noted that the majority of studies indicate that there is no consistent pattern in sex differences in well-being for older persons. Larson conducted a comprehensive review of the literature of the past thirty years on older people's subjective well-being, and stated that, of all the factors considered, health is the one most strongly related to subjective well-being.

Life Satisfaction and Health

The terms "life satisfaction" and "well-being" are often used interchangeably in the literature. Although it could be argued that they are not conceptually the same, to the extent that a higher degree of perceived life-satisfaction maintains a reciprocal relationship with a greater sense of overall well-being, certain comparisons can be made.

Much of the literature on life satisfaction contains measures similar to ones used in the present study, and is, therefore, of interest. Clemente and Sauer [32] found that race and perceived health are the most salient predictors of satisfaction, with whites showing considerably higher scores than blacks, and those with higher self-ratings of health having higher scores. They found that socioeconomic status (SES) indicators have negligible effect on life satisfaction, and they did not find an inverse relationship between age and life satisfaction.

The literature on the relationship between age and life satisfaction is interesting in the lack of consistency and consensus generated by the findings. From their examination of the literature on the subject, Riley and Foner [33] concluded that life satisfaction tends to decline with age. Ten years later, however, it is impossible to draw such a neat and definitive conclusion about the direction of the relationship. The Clemente and Sauer study [32] arrived at the opposite estimation of the nature of the association between age and life satisfaction, as did studies conducted by Edwards and Klemmack [34] and Palmore and Luikart [35]. As noted, when Spreitzer and Snyder's sample was disaggregated by sex, they observed a change in the level of life satisfaction after age sixty-five.

Some discrepancies in research findings are also seen when the literature on sociodemographic factors is examined. Edwards and Klemmack, and Palmore and Luikart observed that family income is an important determinant of life satisfaction. Spreitzer and Snyder and Clemente and Sauer, on the other hand, attributed little strength to SES factors in predicting life satisfaction. In the great majority of studies, race displayed a consistent pattern, with whites indicating higher levels of life satisfaction. In virtually every study in which perceived-health status was used, it proved to be an important determinant of life satisfaction [34, 35, 36, 26]. By extension, it may be postulated that perceived-health status may be a perfect indicator to reflect the general health status of the population.

Disability and Functional Incapacity

A disabling condition is defined as an anatomical or physical abnormality that limits work ability or regular routines and activities of daily living (for example, bathing, dressing, transferring, walking, and other self-care activities). The degree of disability is generally measured by the extent to which an individual can function independently without human assistance. Previous research has shown that the relationship between general health and functional limitations is complicated by the variations in social, demographic, psychological, and cultural characteristics of the population. For instance, several studies have found that people who have the same condition may not necessarily be incapacitated to the same extent, whereas those who have the same level of limitation due to health reasons may be afflicted with different disabling conditions [37, 38, 39]. Furthermore, the diagnostic condition was not considered a strong predictor of the severity of the disability. This finding has cast some doubt on the validity of using only the diagnostic classification of illness or disease as a criterion to determine the degree of functional incapacity or disability.

Chappell [40] has empirically examined the reliability and validity of three measures of the health of the elderly in Manitoba, Canada. Three subsamples were randomly selected from residents living in conventional housing in the community, in subsidized housing, and in institutions providing some form of medical care. The results show that: (1) the Index of Living Skills measures heavy and light tasks; (2) Shanas's Index of Disability [23] is a reliable and valid instrument by which to identify functional incapacities in those living in the community and in institutions, but not in those living in subsidized housing; and (3) the index of chronic conditions (based upon a list of diagnostic categories) is relatively unreliable in all three subgroups of elderly studied.

Basing the information on the first-wave data from the LRHS, Wan [6] presents evidence to show that the sociomedical health indicators (that is, functional limitations and disability measures) are better explanatory variables of perceived health status than socioeconomic and psychological indicators of well-being. He further suggests that the payoff in health status research on index construction is most likely to come from emphasis on measures of physical functional incapacities of disabilities.

A Model of General Health

Health is a multi-dimensional concept, and many conceptual and methodological issues complicate its practical use as a descriptor of the quality of life. The present study aims to formulate a global model in which health is conceptualized as a state of well-being measured by subjective assessment of overall health and life satisfaction, and by physical functional capacities of older adults in a selected study sample derived from the Longitudinal Retirement History Study.

The model consists of three interrelated dimensions of health, physical, mental, and social well-being. These three dimensions are unobserved components of health that can be measured by global indicators of disability level, life satisfaction, and self-assessed health of the study population. A multiple-indicators approach can be applied to identify the structural and measurement model of general health in a panel-study design (see figure 3-1).

This model specifies that the level of functional disability is negatively related to subjectively assessed health (indicator of mental well-being) and life satisfaction (indicator of social well-being), and that life satisfaction is positively associated with subjectively assessed health. The concept of health can be operationally measured by these three dimensions of well-being. However, it is imperative to validate each of these dimensions measured by health indicators before constructing an aggregate index of health. The validation of health indicators as measures of each dimension of well-being is performed in the following sections.

Analysis of Panel Data

Health-status variables included self-assessed health, overall life satisfaction, and functional capacity. Information about physical health was obtained from the responses to the following health-related questions: (1) Is your health better, worse, or the same as that of other people your age? (2)

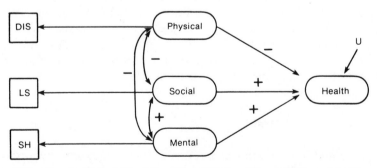

Note: DIS = functional disability; LS = life satisfaction SH = self-assessed health.
Figure 3-1. Multiple Indicators Model of Health

Do you have any health condition, physical handicap, or disability that limits how well you get around? (3) Does your health limit the kind or amount of work or housework you can do? (4) Do you have to stay in your house or in bed all or most of the time? (5) Are you usually able to go outside your home without help from another person? (6) Are you able to use buses, trains or other public transportation without help from others?

Self-assessed health was determined by the response to Question one: those who perceived their health worse than others of their age were assigned a score of 1, and others were assigned a score of 0. As an indicator of psychological well-being, life satisfaction was determined by the response to the following questions: Generally, how satisfied are you with the way you are living now? Those who were unsatisfied with their life were assigned a score of 1, while others were assigned a score of 0.

Functional capacity is defined as the level of dysfunctioning due to physical disability and its resultant dependency on assistance. In this research, functional capacity or incapacity is based upon the responses to questions 2–6 noted above. Two dimensions of functioning level were identified. One indicates the severity of disability, including severe disability (unable to perform work), moderate disability (health limits the kind or amount of work), and no disability. Another dimension represents the dependency level, which includes severe dependency (housebound or bedridden), moderate dependency (requires human assistance for transportation or going outside the home), and no dependency.

Correlations of Three Indicators

In order to examine the relationships of the three indicators, we performed a correlation analysis of three health variables in three waves of LRHS data. The sample was restricted to a total of 4,053 people. The deletion of cases with any missing information from all three waves of the data ensures that all the coefficients are derived from the same cases; otherwise, the interpretation of correlation coefficients would have to be confined to the analysis of a single wave of the panel data.

Table 3–1 presents a correlation matrix of three indicators of health. Self-assessed health (SH) is positively associated with life satisfaction (LS). Their correlations in three waves (1971, 1973, and 1975) of the panel population are .20, .49, and .56, respectively. This finding shows that the strength of the SH-LS relationship increases when the panel group ages. The disability level (DIS) is inversely related to SH and to LS variables, while it has a stronger relation to SH than to LS. Furthermore, this association increases as the panel population ages. These findings imply that functional disability or incapacity may have stronger influence on perceived health than on life satisfaction of the elderly.

Table 3-1
Correlation Matrix of Indicators of Health

Variable[b]	SH71	LS71	DIS71	SH73	LS73	DIS73	SH75	LS75	DIS75
SH71	1.00								
LS71	.20*	1.00							
DIS71	-.45*	-.17*	1.00						
SH73	.46*	.14*	-.38*	1.00					
LS73	.27*	.33*	-.29*	.49*	1.00				
DIS73	-.34*	-.13*	.47*	-.61*	-.44*	1.00			
SH75	.32*	.10*	-.27*	.50*	.33*	-.44*	1.00		
LS75	.20*	.25*	-.20*	.35*	.49*	-.34*	.56*	1.00	
DIS75	-.23*	-.10*	.31*	-.43*	-.34*	.50*	-.69*	-.59*	1.00

$N = 4053$[a]

[a]Those who had incomplete information on health measures in the three waves of LRH study were excluded from this table.
[b]Variables include self-assessed health (SH), life satisfaction (LS), and disability (DIS) for three waves of LRHS data (1971, 1973, and 1975).
*Significant at .05 or lower level.

Health Indicator Models for Panel Data

The multiple-indicator approach employs several indicators of unmeasured concept (unobserved variables, for example, health) to measure the same construct over time. The path linking the unobserved variable with the indicator is called the epistemic correlation or is the square root of the reliability coefficient [41]. The conventional procedure in estimating the reliability coefficient is based on the test-retest correlation, assuming the time variable is perfectly stable over time. In the present study, we use a three-wave, one-indicator model to estimate the reliability and stability coefficients. There are three observed correlations (r_{12}, r_{23}, r_{13}) and three parameters (a, b, and c) to estimate. The model assumes that the reliability coefficient is the same throughout three waves; therefore, this model is identified and a single estimate for each parameter is possible (see figure 3-2).

This model is independently applied to panel data for deriving estimates of reliability and stability measures for three distinct health indicators (self-assessed health, life satisfaction, and disability level). The results are presented in figure 3-3, 3-4, 3-5 and in table 3-2. The over-time correlations for each indicator-variable show that the size of the observed correlations across the three waves of data is moderate and statistically significant, ranging from .32 to .50 for SH, .25 to .49 for LS, and .31 to .50 for DIS.

Columns two, four, and six of table 3-2 give the estimates of stability coefficients across the three waves of panel data. There are two points to be made about these estimates. First, the stability coefficients represent significant increases over the observed correlations among the indicators and reveal that the assessment of general health does not change much over a four-year period. Second, the estimates of stability coefficients are slightly higher for SH and for DIS as compared to those for LS estimates. Furthermore, it is interesting to note that the health variable measured by LS is less reliable than that measured by SH or by DIS indicators.

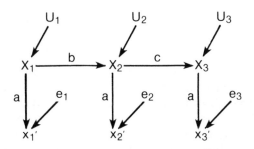

Figure 3-2. Three-Wave, One-Indicator Model

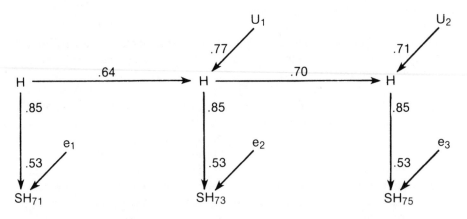

Figure 3-3. Three-Wave, One Health-Indicator Model for Self-Assessed
Health (SH)

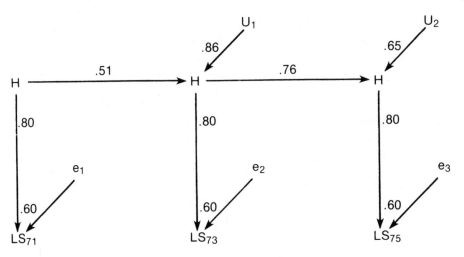

Figure 3-4. Three-Wave, One Health-Indicator Model for Life Satisfaction (LS)

These findings have provided some important evidence on the adequacy
of health indicators in measuring general health as an unmeasured variable.
Moreover, the analysis of the three-wave, one-indicator model shows that
the construct of health is relatively stable, but that its random-measurement
errors remain to be identified through the application of an advanced-multi-
ple indicators model developed by Joreskog and Sorbom [18].

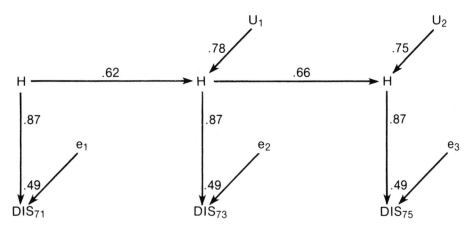

Figure 3-5. Three-Wave, One Health-Indicator Model for Disability Level (DIS)

Predictive Validity of Health Indicators

Predictive validity is concerned with the association of the relevant measure of health with a future criterion. This measurement validation is based on correlating the measure in question with validity variables such as stressful life events, mortality status, and use of health services in the panel-study design. In addition, these validity variables can be regressed on the health indicators so that the causal effect of prior health status on mortality and health-services use can be determined.

In the present study, our analysis is limited to only three waves (1971, 1973, 1975) of LRHS data. The health indicators observed in 1971 are considered as predictor variables or validity variables measured in 1973. Similarly, health indicators measured in 1973 are used to predict the validity variables in 1975. The results of correlation analysis are presented in table 3-3. As we expected, health status measured by three health indicators was significantly associated with validity variables. The self-assessed-health and life-satisfaction scales were inversely related to life stress, mortality, and use of health services, while the disability level was positively related to the validity of the three health indicators. In order to further show the predictive power of these indicators, we performed a panel regression analysis in which the dependent variable (for example, self-assessed health) is regressed on the initial health status (that is, a lagged variable), stressful life events score, and sociodemographic variables. The detailed findings can be found in chapter 7.

Table 3–2
Stability and Reliability Estimates for Three Health Indicators, 1971–1975

| | | | | Health Indicators | | | |
| | SH | | LS | | DIS | |
Time Period	Observed r	Stability Coefficient	Observed r	Stability Coefficient	Observed r	Stability Coefficient
Time-span correlations						
1971–1973	.46	.64	.33	.51	.47	.62
1973–1975	.50	.70	.49	.76	.50	.66
1971–1975	.32	.45	.25	.39	.31	.41
Reliabilities						
1971		.72		.64		.76
1973		.72		.64		.76
1975		.72		.64		.76

SH = self-assessed health; LS = life satisfaction; DIS = disability level.

Table 3-3
The Relationships of Health Indicators to Validity Variables

Validity Variables	Self-Assessed Health	Life Satisfaction	Disability Level
1971–1973 period:		Health in 1971	
Stressful life events[a]	− .13*	− .11*	.21*
Mortality rate	− .39*	− .11*	.44*
Number of physician visits in 1972	− .07*	− .03*	.06*
Number of hospital days in 1972	− .05*	− .00	.05*
1973–1975 period:		Health in 1973	
Stressful life events	− .24*	− .21*	.27*
Mortality rate	− .39*	− .35*	.40*
Number of physician visits in 1974	− .12*	− .06*	.13*
Number of hospital days in 1972	− .04*	− .03*	.04*

*Significant at .05 or lower level.
[a]Weighted scores for life-change events were constructed.

References

1. Belloc, N.B., L. Breslow, and J.R. Hochstein, "The Measurement of Physical Health in a General Population Survey," *American Journal of Epidemiology* 93 (1971):328–336.

2. Hunt, S.M., and J. McEwen, "The Development of a Subjective Health Indicator," *Sociology of Health and Illness* 2 (1980):231–246.

3. Hessler, R.M., et al., "Demographic Context, Social Interaction, and Perceived Health Status," *Journal of Health and Social Behavior* 12 (1971):191–199.

4. Maddox, G.L., "Self-Assessment of Health Status, A Longitudinal Study of Selected Elderly Subjects," *Journal of Chronic Diseases* 17 (1964):449–460.

5. Linn, M.W., "Studies in Rating the Physical, Mental and Social Dysfunction of the Chronically Ill Aged," *Medical Care* 14 (1976):119–125.

6. Wan, T.T.H., "Predicting Self-Assessed Health Status: A Multivariate Approach," *Health Services Research* 11 (1976):464–477.

7. Katz, S., and C.A. Akdom, "A Measure of Primary Sociological Function," *International Journal of Health Services* 6 (1976):493–506.

8. Kahn, R.L., et al., "Brief Objective Measures for the Determination of Mental Status in the Aged," *American Journal of Psychiatry* 107 (1960):326–328.

9. Williams, R.G., et al., "Disability: A Model and Measurement Technique," *British Journal of Preventive and Social Medicine* 30 (1976): 71–78.

10. Maklan, C., C.F. Cannell, and J.R.P. French, "Subjective and Objective Concepts of Health: A Background Statement for Research," unpublished paper, (Ann Arbor: Institute for Social Research, University of Michigan, 1974).

11. Campbell, A., P. Converse, and W.L. Rogers, *The Quality of American Life* (New York: Russell Sage Foundation, 1976).

12. Andrews, F.M., and S.N. Withey, "Developing Measures of Perceived Life Quality: Results From Several National Surveys," *Social Indicators Research* 1 (1974):1–26.

13. Reynolds, W.J., W.A. Rushing, and D.L. Miles, "The Validation of a Functional Status Index," *Journal of Health and Social Behavior* 15 (1974):271–288.

14. Ware, J.E., A.R. Davies, and R.H. Brook, *Conceptualization and Measurement of Health for Adults in the Health Insurance Study: Vol. VI. Analysis for Relationships Among Health Status Measures* (Santa Monica, Cal.: The Rand Corporation, 1980).

15. Althauser, R.P., and T.A. Heberlein, "A Causal Assessment of Validity and the Multitrait-Multimethod Matrix," in E.F. Borgatta and G.W. Bohrnstedt, eds., *Sociological Methodology,* (San Francisco: Jossey-Bass, Inc., 1970).

16. Althauser, R.P., "Inferring Validity From the Multitrait-Multimethod Matrix: Another Assessment," in Hil, Costner, eds. *Sociological Methodology* (San Francisco: Jossey-Bass, Inc., 1974).

17. Werts, C.E. and R.N. Linn, "Cautions in Applying Various Procedures for Determining the Reliability and Validity of Multiple-Item Scales," *American Sociological Review* 35 (1970):757–759.

18. Joreskog, K.G., and D. Sorbom. "Statistical Models and Methods for Analysis of Longitudinal Data," in D.J. Aigner and A.S. Goldberger, eds., *Latent Variables in Socioeconomic Models* (Amsterdam: North-Holland, 1977).

19. Berry, D.C., J.W. Bush, and R.M. Kaplan, Testing for Variations in Social Group Preferences for Function Levels of a Health Index, (paper presented at the annual meeting of the American Statistical Association) August 1975.

20. Bergner, M. et al., "The Sickness Impact Profile: Validation of a Health Status Measure," *Medical Care* 14 (1976):57–67.

21. Pollard, W.E., et al., "The Sickness Impact Profile: Reliability of Health Status Measure," *Medical Care* 14 (1976):146–155.

22. Shanas, E., and G. Maddox, "Aging, Health and Organizations of Health Resources, in R. Bingstock and E. Shanas, eds., *Handbook of Aging and Social Science* (New York: Van Nostrand-Reinhold, 1976).

23. Shanas, E., "Health Status of Older People: Cross National Implications," *American Journal of Public Health* 3 (1974):261–264.

24. Maddox, G.L., and E.B. Douglass, "Aging and Individual Differences: A Longitudinal Analysis of Social, Psychological, and Physiological Indicators," *Journal of Gerontology* 29 (1974):555-563.

25. Kovar, M.D., "Health of the Elderly and Use of Health Services," *Public Health Reports* 92 (1977):109-129.

26. Spreitzer, E., and E. Snyder, "Correlates of Life Satisfaction Among the Aged," *Journal of Gerontology* 29 (1974):454-459.

27. Palmore, E., "The Effects of Aging on Activities and Attitudes," *Gerontologist* 8 (1968):259-263.

28. Streib, G., and C. Schneider, *Retirement in American Society* (Ithaca, N.Y.: Cornell University Press, 1971).

29. Verbrugge, L.M., "Females and Illness: Recent Trends in Sex Differences in the United States," *Journal of Health and Social Behavior* 17 (1976):387-407.

30. Nathanson, C.A., "Sex, Illness, and Medical Care: A Review of Data, Theory, and Method," *Social Science and Medicine* 11 (1977):13-25.

31. Larson, R., "Thirty Years of Research on the Subjective Well-Being of Older Americans," *Journal of Gerontology* 33 (1978):109-129.

32. Clemente, F., and W. Sauer, "Life Satisfaction in the United States," *Social Forces* 54 (1976):621-631.

33. Riley, M., and A. Foner, *Aging and Society, Vol. 1.* (New York: Russell Sage Foundation, 1968).

34. Edwards, J.N., and D.L. Klemmack, "Correlates of Life Satisfaction: A Reexamination," *Journal of Gerontology* 28 (1973):497-502.

35. Palmore, E., and C. Luikart, "Health and Social Factors Related to Life Satisfaction," *Journal of Health and Social Behavior* 13 (1971): 68-80.

36. Tornstam, L., "Health and Self-Perception: A Systems Theoretical Approach," *Gerontologist* 15 (1975):264-270.

37. Haber, L.D., "Disabling Effects of Chronic Disease or Impairment," *Journal of Chronic Diseases* 24 (1971):469-487.

38. Wan, T.T.H., "Correlates and Consequence of Severe Disabilities," *Journal of Occupational Medicine* 16 (1976):234-244.

39. Taylor, P.L., and A.J. Fairrie, "Chronic Disabilities and Capacity for Work," *British Journal of Preventative and Social Medicine* 22 (1968): 86-93.

40. Chappell, N.C., "Measuring Functional Ability and Chronic Health Conditions Among the Elderly: A Research Note on the Adequacy of Three Instruments," *Journal of Health and Social Behavior* 22 (1981): 90-102.

41. Sullivan, J.L., and S. Feldman, *Multiple Indicators: An Introduction* (Beverly Hills: Sage Publications, 1979).

4 Role Loss as a Stressful Event in Later Life

This chapter focuses on major role losses that are common to the life experience of the elderly. In our conceptual framework, roles are defined as rights, duties, and expectations that are attached to positions in society. It is well-known that age is inversely related to the number of positions held.

Common role losses in old age include loss of the roles or *worker* (primarily through retirement), *spouse* (through widowhood, divorce, or separation) and *parent* (through the departure of children from the family). It should be noted that, while the losses of worker and spouse roles are *discrete* role losses, the loss of the parent role actually involves a progressive loss, since parental responsibilities decrease as children mature. The present study deals only with the loss of the parental role by a discrete measure of departure of the children.

Related Research

In order to realize the impact of major role losses on health care and use of health services, the meaning of these lifetime roles must be understood. The spouse role is characterized as an informal role with both instrumental and expressive functions. Nye has defined eight tasks of the role of marriage partner: housekeeper, provider, child socializer, therapeutic sounding-board, community liaison, kinship provider, and sexual and recreational partner [1]. While some of these tasks decrease in importance with aging, the crisis of a spouse's death, which Hill [2] terms the crisis of dismemberment, is still disorganizing to the survivor. Lopata [3], studying 300 Chicago widows, observed that death disrupts the life pattern of the surviving spouse, necessitating a reorganization of roles. The loss of a partner can imply a personal loss of someone with whom experiences were shared, as well as a change of life style and social relations outside the conjugal unit. Identity loss also accompanies widowhood to the degree that the individual identifies with the spouse role [4,5].

There is controversy over whether widowhood is more disruptive to the lives of men or women. Those emphasizing expressive aspects of the role argue that men are more disadvantaged because they have previously relied on their wives to maintain liaisons with family, friends, and community [6].

Others, stressing instrumental functions, counter that men have advantages in maintaining participation because they experience less income loss and are usually self-reliant for transportation [7].

Research indicates that divorce (or separation) is at least as disruptive to the lives of older people as widowhood [8, 9]. It should be pointed out that the absence of rituals attached to divorce and the lack of support offered to the divorced person, as compared to the widowed, may make this a more disruptive experience at any stage in the life cycle. While the divorced represent only about 2 percent of the aged population, societal trends would lead us to expect that the proportion of divorced persons will increase with each successive age cohort; therefore, attention must also be directed to this form of role loss.

The parental role is also an informal social role. Research suggests that, while this role is not lost with advancing age, its content does change. Emphasis changes from needs provision and financial support to emotional support. The departure of the children from the household may be a key event, altering the content of the parental role. The general availability of children to both give and receive emotional support after their departure from the household is well-documented. Eighty percent of old people in the United States have at least one surviving child and 75 percent share a household with a child or live within thirty minutes of a child [10]. As is true of current childbearing trends, working-class elderly have more children than do middle-class families.[11].

Considered a formal role, the work role has both instrumental and expressive tasks. As workers communicate with each other, work may be a basis for social relations. Blau [4] has noted that the retired person may be deprived of the common experience that is shared by people who work. Like widowhood, retirement may entail loss of identity and reorganization of roles as well as a change in social relations. At a minimum, retirement requires reorganization of time. Unlike widowhood, however, loss of the work role does not necessarily have a negative connotation. For some it may bring a release from boring or frustrating work. Perhaps in retirement more clearly than in widowhood, an individual's preparation for the event, attitude toward the role and ability to substitute roles of kin, friend, or organization member may affect his ease of adjustment.

In current literature, retirement has been treated primarily as a male adjustment, under the assumption that work roles are secondary and not of major importance to females. Consequently, sex differences in adaptation are just beginning to be explored [12, 13].

There is reason to suspect that major-role losses as change events may do more than simply happen concurrently with other life changes of advancing age. These role losses may actually be directly related to each other and to the occurrence of other life changes of lesser magnitude.

Alterations in income have been clearly linked to major-role losses. Income loss even to the degree described as poverty has been associated with widowhood and retirement [7, 14, 15, 16]. Loss of means of transportation and an increased residential mobility have also been associated with loss of spouse [7, 17]. Perhaps reflecting the foregoing variables, changes in life satisfaction resulting in lowered satisfaction are associated with widowhood and retirement [15, 16, 18].

To date, the causal relationship between major-role losses and changes in health status and use of health services remains obscure. Part of the difficulty in determining the causal relationship between role loss and health status stems from the intercorrelation of these factors, particularly with regard to psychological well-being. As Eckenrode and Gore [19] have noted, the loss of informal roles, such as spouse or parent, may contribute to deterioration of the psychological state. Conversely, deterioration of the psychological state may contribute to the loss of the roles of spouse or worker. The latter explanation may have particular salience for divorced persons. This problem is exacerbated by the cross-sectional design of most recent studies, which limits ability to determine temporal sequence of events in the causal chain. The current research aims to overcome this deficit by employing panel data for analysis.

The effect of major-role losses on health may be cumulative, since loss of two or more roles simultaneously may create added deteriorative effects. However, the independent effects of major-role losses on health are not conclusive. Research has also shown that being married facilitates adjustment to retirement. Married and never-married people have higher morale than the divorced and widowed [20, 21] in retirement.

Niemi [22] has noted higher mortality in the short term among retirees whose wives died, but no effects on mortality in the long run. There is some evidence that the widowed, particularly men, experience poor mental health as shown by a higher rate of suicide and mental disorder [23, 24].

Maddison and Viola [25] discovered that there were more complaints about health in widows between the ages of forty-five and fifty-nine-years than among a comparable nonbereaved group. Heyman and Gianturco [26], however, have refuted such claims, finding in a longitudinal study that widowed people experience only time-related health deterioration. Likewise, Elwell and Maltbie-Crannell [15] concluded that the effect of widowhood on subjective health assessment was indirect, mediated through income status.

The effects of the departure of children from the household on the health of the elderly have not been investigated. One reason for neglect of this subject is that such departure usually takes place in middle age, not old age. Evidence to date does indicate that the impact of the so-called empty-nest syndrome has been overstated. Lowenthal and Chiroboga [27] found that the period following the launching of the last child was not stressful. In fact, middle-aged women whose children were launched reported more positive self-concepts than did women whose children remained at home. For this reason, we suspect that the departure of children will either have no impact or have a positive effect on health [28].

The causal nature of the relationship between retirement and health status is difficult to identify because retirement may occur as a direct consequence of poor health. It is well known that health problems are one of the major factors precipitating a withdrawal from the labor force [29-36]. In fact, in analyzing the first wave of data from LRHS data, Schwab [35] found that 65 percent of men aged fifty-eight to sixty-three years who were already retired in 1969 cited health as their main reason for labor-force withdrawal. Kimmel, Price, and Walker [37] report that health status and preretirement feelings are the strongest predictors of retirement attitudes.

In order to ascertain the causal relationship between retirement and health status in our study, we excluded those who were in poor health in the beginning of the study from our analysis (see chapter 1).

To date, the effect of retirement on health is ambiguous. Studies that control for health at the time of retirement have generally found very little impact of retirement on physical or mental health [28]. However, Thompson [16] has noted an association between retirement and subjective health observing that assessment of health was an intervening factor in determining morale among retired, but not working, men. Kimmel, Price, and Walker [37] have also observed that those who had more positive attitudes about retirement and who expressed greater satisfaction with retirement also had better health status. In this case, health status may be a function of whether retirement was voluntary or involuntary.

Although most of the evidence indicates that retirement does not have a direct impact on health, a recent retrospective study [38] of 1,136 married white men indicated that, after controlling for age and history of hospitalization for myocardial infarction, retirees had an 80 percent greater risk of death from heart attacks. These data suggest that retirement and subsequent mortality may be linked. To date, there are few studies such as ours that control for health status at the time of retirement in order to determine the impact of this major-role loss on health and health-service utilization. From the available literature, it appears that loss of the spouse role has a greater impact than does retirement in the above areas. Nonetheless, our prospective study design, which controls for health and retirement status in the beginning of our study, should increase our understanding of the effects of the loss of work role. The results of the analysis of the Longitudinal Retirement History Survey data are presented in the following sections.

Analysis of Panel Data

Differentials in the Experience of a Major-Role Loss

Table 4-1 displays the proportion and number of persons who experienced a major-role loss for each of the three periods of our study (1969-1971, 1971-1973, 1973-1975) and for the entire six-year study period. As expected, retirement was the event most frequently experienced during the entire study period. Finally, 70.5 percent of respondents who were working in 1969 retired during the subsequent six years. Almost another 10 percent (9.6 percent) who were married in 1969 were widowed during the following six years. Divorce and separation occurred to a lesser degree during this period. Two percent of the population experienced this event. It should be noted that this figure is compatible with the proportion of divorced and separated elderly in the nation as a whole, which is also 2 percent [39].

A closer look at table 4-1 reveals the proportion of elderly who experience each of the five events during each of the periods studied. The variation in the likelihood of major-role losses occurring in different periods of our study probably reflects the advancing age of the cohort and the variations in composition of our sample due to attrition and mortality. As shown, retirement was experienced by a greater proportion of the study population during the second period, when respondents were between the ages of sixty and sixty-seven years. However, no substantial differences in

Table 4-1

Proportion and Number of Persons in the Prospective Study Sample Who Experienced Major Role Losses, 1969-1975

Role Loss	1969-1975 (N = 5,883)	1969-1971 (N = 5,332)	1971-1973 (N = 5,053)	1973-1975 (N = 4,748)
Retirement	70.5 (4,149)	24.2 (1,289)	31.7 (1,604)	26.5 (1,256)
Widowhood	9.6 (562)	2.3 (121)	3.4 (171)	5.7 (270)
Divorce	0.8 (45)	0.1 (6)	0.2 (9)	0.6 (30)
Separation	1.8 (108)	0.2 (10)	1.5 (77)	0.4 (21)
Departure of children from home	22.1 (1,023)	2.8 (151)	19.0 (959)	0.3 (13)

the proportion of persons experiencing this event during each of the periods of this study were observed.

Widowhood and divorce, on the other hand, were most likely to occur when respondents reached the ages of sixty-two and sixty-nine years. Separation most often occurred when respondents were somewhat younger, between the ages of sixty and sixty-seven years (period two).

The event of departure of the children shows the most variation by time period. While 19 percent of the population experienced this event when they were between the ages of sixty and sixty-seven years, only 2.8 percent and 3 percent of our sample experienced departure of the children in the first and third study periods, respectively.

Table 4-2 examines the relative importance of several sociodemographic explanatory variables (age, race/sex, occupation, and education) in the retirement process during the three study periods. Data in this table show occupation, followed by age, is clearly the most important predictor of the decision to retire. Race/sex and education, while of lesser importance, were significant-but-weak predictors in period one (1969-1971) but not in subsequent study periods.

The fact that occupation has a strong effect on early retirement deserves closer inspection. Four occupational categories were considered: white-collar, blue-collar, service, and farm occupations. There appears to be considerable variation in the decision to retire among occupational categories. Service workers were the most likely to retire during the period between 1969-1971 when all respondents were comparatively younger. During successive periods, however, blue-collar and white-collar workers were more likely to retire, with the greatest amount of retirement occurring for white-collar workers during the last period of our study—when respondents reached sixty-two to sixty-nine years. The fewer physical demands placed on workers in white-collar employment may explain their tendency to retire at later ages.

Advancing age is also related to the occurrence of retirement. Respondents who were comparatively older (aged sixty-two and sixty-three in 1969) were more likely to retire during the first period of the study, 1969-1971. These respondents and the next younger group (aged sixty to sixty-one) were more likely to retire in the second study period, 1971-1973. It should be noted that, during this period, respondents who were sixty-two or sixty-three years old in 1969 were between the ages of sixty-four and sixty-five years. The youngest respondents in our sample (aged fifty-eight and fifty-nine years) were the most likely to retire during the last period of our study. At this time (period three), these respondents were between the ages of sixty-two and sixty-five years. Our data shows a pronounced tendency to retire at around the age of sixty-five in each of the time periods studied.

Table 4-2
Unadjusted (P) and Adjusted (P′) Proportions of Persons Who Became Retirees in the Prospective Study Sample, 1969–1975

	Percentage of Workers Who Became Retirees in Each Period					
	1969–1971		*1971–1973*		*1973–1975*	
Characteristics in 1969	P	P′	P	P′	P	P′
Age (Beta)	(.22)*		(.12)*		(.15)*	
58–59	11	14	26	24	33	32
60–61	26	26	35	34	27	27
62–63	42	37	35	37	15	16
Race-Sex	(.07)*		(.01)ns		(.03)ns	
White male	22	24	33	31	27	26
Nonwhite male	22	18	27	29	30	30
White female	31	28	30	32	25	24
Nonwhite female	34	13	23	32	24	28
Occupation	(.52)*		(.24)*		(.10)*	
White-Collar	7	6	33	35	31	30
Blue-Collar	6	8	46	46	30	28
Service	54	53	19	18	20	20
Farm	17	18	26	25	28	27
Education	(.04)*		(.06)*		(.02)ns	
0–8th grade	27	22	33	34	24	25
9–12th grade	24	25	32	31	27	27
College	19	26	27	25	29	27

*The net effect of an explanatory variable on retirement is statistically significant at .05 or lower level.
ns: not statistically significant.

The race/sex variable was only significant in the first study period
(1969–1971). A greater tendency to retire at a relatively early age was found
among white females and nonwhite males. Nonwhite females were least apt
to retire.

Differences in educational level, while significant for the periods
1969–1971 and 1971–1973, were not substantial. Perhaps the only trend
worth pointing out is the tendency of those with eighth-grade or lower
educational attainments to retire between the ages of sixty to sixty-seven.
The data tend to support our previous conclusion that service and blue-
collar employment require less education but are more physically demanding, and, therefore, may force earlier retirement.

Concomitance of Major-Role Losses

Having examined the frequencies with which major-role losses occurred in
our population and sociodemographic differentials in retirement, we address the next question in our analysis: what is the extent to which major-
role losses are related? Table 4–3 reveals the correlations between major-
role losses in each of the three study periods. During the period from
1969–1971, retirement was significantly correlated to widowhood and the
departure of children from the family. Departure of children was also
significantly related to widowhood and divorce.

During the second (1971–1973) and third (1973–1975) study periods,
retirement was correlated to separation. Retirement was also significantly
related to departure of the children between 1971–1973. It is worth noting
that in these successive periods of our study, none of the other major role
losses studied were significantly related.

To summarize our data focusing upon retirement, it is apparent that
there is little evidence of the concomitance of major role losses. No clear
pattern of events associated with retirement emerges. Retirement was
associated with the experiencing of widowhood when our sample as a whole
was comparatively younger (fifty-eight to sixty-three). Perhaps, experiencing this event relatively early in life contributes to change in life style and
consequently to a decision to retire. Another explanation might be that illness of a spouse leads to a decision to retire at a relatively early age in order
to be a caregiver.

There also appears to be an association between the events of retirement and departure of the children from the family during the first two
periods of our study, when the study population as a whole was comparatively younger.

The data in table 4–3 portray a somewhat static picture of the relation
of events in each of the periods studied. Little evidence of the concomitance

Table 4–3

Correlation Matrix of Major-Role Losses in Each Period, 1969–1975

	Retired	Widowed	Divorced	Separated	Children Departed
1969–1971 (N = 5,332)					
Retirement	1.00				
Widowhood	.06*	1.00			
Divorce	− .01	− .01	1.00		
Separation	− .00	− .01	− .00	1.00	
Departure of children	.04*	.06*	.03*	− .00	1.00
1971–1973 (N = 5,053)					
Retirement	1.00				
Widowhood	.02	1.00			
Divorce	− .02	− .00	1.00		
Separation	− .04*	− .02	− .00	1.00	
Departure of children	.04*	− .01	− .00	.01	1.00
1973–1975 (N = 4,748)					
Retirement	1.00				
Widowhood	.02	1.00			
Divorce	.00	− .02	1.00		
Separation	.04*	− .02	− .01	1.00	
Departure of children	− .01	.02	− .00	− .00	1.00

*Significant at 0.05 or lower level.

of retirement and other major-role losses is revealed in these tables. This finding implies that the role losses studied may be independent events that occur in later life.

Effect of Role Losses on Perceived Health

To clearly identify a causal relationship, we traced the health consequences of retirement and other major-role losses over the entire study period. The dependent variable, personal perception of health status, was determined by the respondents' assessments of how their health compared with that of others of the same age. A dichotomized health variable is used. People who perceived their health as being worse than that of others were coded as 1, and those who perceived their health as being the same or better than that of others were coded as 0. Independent variables included five role-loss variables measured in the three study periods (1969–1971, 1971–1973, and 1973–1975). Data in table 4–4 show that role loss resulting from retirement had an adverse effect on health in 1971, but not in the later periods. The most striking result is that widowhood was the strongest role-loss variable

Table 4–4
Regression Analysis of the Likelihood of Illness of Those with Perceived Poor Health, by Role Losses and Survey Year

Role Losses in a Period[a]	1971		1973		1975	
	B	Beta	B	Beta	B	Beta
Retirement	.08*	.12	.00	.00	.12	.00
Widowhood	.53*	.29	.34*	.12	6.02*	.14
Divorce	− .07	− .01	.17	.01	− 1.13	− .01
Separation	.06	.01	.08	.02	− .65	− .00
Departure of children	.03	.02	.02	.02	4.50*	.12
Constant	.05		.48		.33	
Mean	.08		.51		.18	
Standard deviation	.27		.50		.38	
R^2	.107		.016		.035	
Total (N)	(5,078)		(4,737)		(4,262)	

[a]Role loss variables are dichotomized: the presence of a role loss in a given period is coded 1, and 0 otherwise.

*Significant at .05 or lower level.

affecting perceived health. This finding has substantiated the fact that widowhood probably is the most devastating life event that will adversely affect the sense of well-being of the elderly.

Panel regression analyses are used to examine the hypothesis that role losses resulting from retirement, change in marital status, and change in parental role through departure of children from home have a significant effect on health status of the elderly. In the panel regression analysis, the dependent variable at Time 2 is regressed on itself (a lagged variable) and the independent variables at Time 1. This analysis is more useful than cross-sectional analysis for generating information about the cause and effect relationship between role loss and health. Furthermore, the gross (under-standardized regression coefficient, B) and net (standardized regression coefficient, Beta) effect of role loss on health variables are shown in this analysis.

Table 4–5 presents panel regression coefficients, with self-assessed health in 1973 being regressed on the role-loss variable (a summated score of the total losses during 1969–1971), the initial level of health status, and

Table 4-5
Panel Regression Coefficients of the Effects of Role Losses (1969–1971) on Self-Assessed Health (1973), by Retirement Status in 1971, Controlling for Prior Health Status and Social Demographic Characteristics

| | Self-Assessed Poor Health in 1973 | | | | | |
| | Total | | Retirees | | Workers | |
Predictors	B	Beta	B	Beta	B	Beta
Role Losses (1969–1971)[a]	.033*	.048	.132*	.097	.067*	.043
Prior Status[b]	.454*	.355	.464*	.432	.440*	.310
Age	− .003	− .019	− .009	− .003	− .001	− .005
SES	− .001*	− .036	.001	.023	− .002*	− 0.56
Sex (male = 1; female = 0)	.037*	.046	.027	.033	.037*	.046
Race (white = 1; nonwhite = 0)	.002	.002	.021	.017	− .006	− .005
Constant	.274		.432		.203	
Mean	.075		.165		.119	
Standard	.263		.372		.324	
R^2	.140		.219		.111	
Total (N)	(5,107)		(1,193)		(3,914)	

[a]The sum of total role losses occurring in 1969–1971.
[b]Status in 1971 was used as a lagged variable in the equation Poor health = 1; Good health = 0.
*Significant at .05 or lower level.

four sociodemographic variables (age, SES, sex and race). The results given in table 4–5 show that role loss has a significant effect on the perception of health, net of prior level of health, and other sociodemographic variables.

One way to test the consistency of this finding is to perform separate regression analyses for retirees and workers. In doing this, we found role losses still exerted a significant positive effect on poor health. These results may reflect an increase in the experience of a variety of role losses, adversely affecting the perception of health of an elderly population.

In order to examine the net effect of role losses during a five-year period (1969–1973) on self-assessed health in 1975, we performed three more regression analyses. Here, we found no significant net effect of this variable on perception of health in the total sample and in the working group. However, among those who were retired in 1973, the role-loss variable has a significant influence on self-assessed health in 1975. This finding has provided further evidence of an adverse effect of retirement on self-assessed health.

Effect of Role Losses on Life Satisfaction

Tables 4-6, 4-7, and 4-8 display the effects of individual role losses and combined-role-loss variables on dissatisfaction with life. Dissatisfaction with life was gauged by a question that required respondents to assess their life satisfaction as compared to others of the same age, over the several time periods studied. Analysis of the data on dissatisfaction proceeded in the same manner as analysis of the effects of role loss on self-assessed health status.

Examination of table 4-6, which shows the effects of five role losses on dissatisfaction, reveals some interesting findings. Most notable is the fact that the experiencing of retirement between 1969-1971 is significantly associated with increased dissatisfaction, while the experiencing of retirement in later periods is not. This finding indicates that those in the cohort studied who experienced retirement at relatively younger ages (between age

Table 4-6

Regression Analysis of the Likelihood of Illness of Those Dissatisfied with Their Lives, by Role Losses and Survey Year

Role Losses in a Given Period	Dissatisfaction of Life					
	1971		1973		1975	
	B	Beta	B	Beta	B	Beta
Retirement	.052*	.068	.012	.015	− .211	− .022
Widowhood	.265*	.122	.644*	.318	.481*	.271
Divorce	.054	.066	− .034	− .004	.014	.003
Separation	.191	.026	− .003	− .001	.248*	.040
Departure of children	.036	.019	− .018	− .019	.045	.006
Constant	.098		.158		.192	
Mean	.118		.170		.215	
Standard deviation	.323		.375		.411	
R²	.022		.102		.075	
Total (N)	(5,386)		(5,107)		(4,748)	

[a]Role loss variables are dichotomized: the presence of a role loss in a given period is coded as 1, and 0 otherwise.

*Significant at .05 or lower level.

Table 4-7
Panel Regression Coefficients of the Effects of Role Losses (1969–1971) on Overall Life Satisfaction (1973), by Retirement Status in 1971, Controlling for the Prior Life-Satisfaction Status and Social Demographic Characteristics

Predictors	Life Dissatisfaction 1973					
	Total		Retirees		Workers	
	B	Beta	B	Beta	B	Beta
Role losses (1969–1971[a])	.059*	.077	.172*	.118	.136*	.077
Prior status	.286*	.245	.281*	.261	.282*	.233
Age	− .006*	− .039	− .017*	.070	.004	.027
SES	− .002*	− .059	− .003*	.064	− .002*	.050
Sex (male = 1; female = 0)	.055*	.062	.079*	.091	.040*	.044
Race (white = 1; nonwhite = 0)	.040*	− .031	− .064	− .048	− .033	− .027
Constant	.585		1,145		.451	
Mean	.170		.194		.162	
Standard deviation	.375		.395		.369	
R²	.081		.119		.072	
Total (N)	(5,107)		(1,193)		(3,914)	

[a]The sum of total role losses occurring in 1969–1971.
[b]Status in 1971 was used as a lagged variable in the equation; Dissatisfaction = 1; Satisfaction = 0.
*Significant at .05 or lower level.

fifty-eight and sixty-three) were more likely to be dissatisfied with life than were those who retired when they were older. In fact, although not significant, the effect of retirement in the last period when respondents were between the ages of sixty-three to sixty-nine years was to reduce dissatisfaction as shown by the negative association.

It should also be observed that widowhood had the most consistent effect on life satisfaction. Respondents who experienced widowhood during each of the periods studied were more likely to report dissatisfaction with their lives; thus widowhood had a negative impact on life satisfaction at all ages. Separation, on the other hand, was associated only with dissatisfaction with life in the last period studied. It may be that the occurrence of this event relatively late in life (when respondents were between the ages of sixty-three and sixty-nine years) contributes to a greater feeling of hopelessness and, therefore, dissatisfaction.

Tables 4–7 and 4–8 show the relative impact of the experience of

Table 4–8
Panel Regression Coefficients of the Effects of Role Losses (1969–1973) on Overall Life Satisfaction (1975), by Retirement Status in 1973; Controlling for the Prior Life-Satisfaction Status and Social Demographic Characteristics

| | Life Dissatisfaction in 1975 | | | | | |
| | Total | | Retirees | | Workers | |
Predictors	B	Beta	B	Beta	B	Beta
Role losses (1969–1973)[a]	.014	.024	.041*	.050	− .019	− .028
Prior status[b]	.378*	.336	.462*	.440	.348*	.301
Age	.004	.023	− .001	− .008	.004	.020
SES	− .002*	− .038	.001	.016	− .001	− .020
Sex (male = 1; female = 0)	.051*	.052	.049*	.055	.037	.038
Race (white = 1; nonwhite = 0)	− .062*	− .045	− .027	− .019	− .017*	− .054
Constant	.016		.068		.006	
Mean	.215		.231		.198	
Standard deviation	.411		.422		.398	
R^2	.128		.210		.099	
Total (N)	(4,748)		(2,450)		(2,298)	

[a]The sum of role losses occurring in 1969–1973.
[b]Status in 1973 was used as a lagged variable in the equation. Dissatisfaction = 1; Satisfaction = 0.
*Significant at .05 or lower level.

cumulative role losses on life satisfaction in 1973 (table 4–7) and 1975 (table 4–8) when controlling for prior satisfaction with life and for several socio-demographic variables. As table 4–7 shows, the experiencing of major role losses between 1969–1971 was significantly related to greater dissatisfaction with life among all groups studied. Among those who had experienced major-role losses, both people who had retired in 1971 and those who were still working had lower life satisfaction in 1973. On the other-hand, the experiencing of major role losses had only a significant effect on life satisfaction among those who were retired in 1973 (table 4–8). A possible explanation for the findings presented in these two tables is that some role losses such as widowhood may be less anticipated at relatively younger ages and, therefore, may have a devastating effect on life satisfaction, regardless of retirement status. However, at later ages the loss of major roles may be anticipated and may lead to greater dissatisfaction with life only when the work role is not available to compensate for other losses.

What is clear from our data in both tables 4-7 and 4-8 is that, among retirees, the loss of major roles at all ages exerted a synergistic effect on dissatisfaction with life.

Effect of Role Losses on Disability Levels

The effect of major role losses on disability level was analyzed by using the same procedure for analysis described previously. As shown in table 4-9, retirement was associated with disability in all three periods studied. The same finding was true of widowhood. None of the other life changes studied (divorce, separation, or departure of the children) was significantly related to functional capacity.

As with our findings for life satisfaction, major-role losses between 1969 and 1971 were associated with greater dissability in 1973 among both retired and nonretired workers. However, major-role losses (between 1969-1973) were associated only with disability among retirees in 1975.

Table 4-9
Regression Analysis of Disability Levels, by Role Losses and Survey Year

	Disability Level					
	1971		1973		1975	
Role Loss in a Given Period[a]	B	Beta	B	Beta	B	Beta
Retirement	.311*	.197	.167*	.092	.055*	− .028
Widowhood	1.437*	.317	1.753*	.373	1.226*	.352
Divorce	− .259	− .013	− .075	.004	.149	.014
Separation	− .161	− .010	.061	.009	.120	.009
Departure of children	.048	.012	− .026	− .012	.224	.014
Constant	.199		.410		.432	
Mean	.307		.501		.493	
Standard deviation	.672		.844		.846	
R^2	.148		.150		.125	
Total (N)	(5,386)		(5,107)		(4,748)	

[a]Role loss variables are dichotomized: the presence of a role loss in a given period is coded as 1, and 0 otherwise.

*Significant at .05 or lower level.

Effect of Role Losses on the Use of Health Services

Our analysis of health-service utilization was confined to the cumulative effects of role losses by retirement status. Utilization was measured by the presence (coded as 1) or absence (coded as 0) of physician visits in 1972 and 1974 (tables 4–10 and 4–11) and by the presence (coded as 1) or absence (coded as 0) of an incidence of hospitalization in 1972 and in 1974. (The years 1972 and 1974 were implied by the wording of the question relating to use of services. These questions asked in 1973 and 1975 referred to the use of services during the preceding year.)

Table 4–10
Panel Regression Coefficients of the Effects of Role Losses (1969–1971) on the Likelihood of Making a Physician Visit (1972), by Retirement Status in 1971, Controlling for the Prior Use, Health-Status Variables, and Social Demographic Characteristics

| | Made a Doctor's Visit in 1972 | | | | | |
| | Total | | Retirees | | Workers | |
Predictors	B	Beta	B	Beta	B	Beta
Role losses (1969–1971)[a]	− .054	− .022	.120	.019	.092	.014
Prior self-assessed health[b]	4.686	.025	4,503	.031	5.001	.023
Prior life satisfaction[b]	2.77	.018	4.689	.035	1.885	.012
Prior disability levels[b]	.870	.011	1.063	.018	1.056	.012
Prior visits[b]	.330*	.330	.331*	.331*	.332*	.332
Age	− .051	− .003	.889	.029	− .066	− .004
SES	.170*	.035	.341*	.076	.134	.027
Sex (male = 1; female = 0)	− 2.971	− .025	− 6.582*	− .060	− 2.031	.017
Race (white = 1; nonwhite = 0)	3.66	.022	− 1.602	− .010	4,871	.029
Constant	28.305		− 41.353			
Mean	52.125		52.221		52.095	
Standard deviation	49.960		49.972		49.963	
R^2	.120		.129		.119	
Total (N)	(5,107)		(1,192)		(3,914)	

[a]The sum of role losses occurring in (1969 – 1971).

[b]Indicators measured in 1971.

*Significant at .05 or lower level.

Table 4–11
Panel Regression Coefficients of the Effects of Role Losses (1969–1973) on the Likelihood of Making a Physician Visit (1974), by Retirement Status in 1973; Controlling for the Prior Use and Health-Status Variables, and Social Demographic Characteristics

| | Made a Doctor's Visit in 1974 | | | | | |
| | Total | | Retirees | | Workers | |
Predictors	B	Beta	B	Beta	B	Beta
Role losses (1967–1973)[a]	.01	.00	.35	.00	− 2.71	− .03
Prior self-assessed health[b]	4.37	.03	3.08	.02	6.28	.03
Prior life satisfaction[b]	− 3.18	− .02	− 2.31	0.02	− 3.90	− .03
Prior disability levels[b]	3.94*	.07	4.75*	.09	2.17	.03
Prior visits[b]	.29*	.30	.30*	.31	.29*	.29
Age	.47	.02	.36	.02	.53	.02
SES	.29*	.06	.19	.04	.37*	.08
Sex (male = 1; female = 0)	− 4.83*	− .04	− 5.23	− .05	− 4.53	− .04
Race (white = 1; nonwhite = 0)	− 5.25	− .03	− 2.98	− .02	− 7.09*	− .04
Constant	4.26		14.21		.26	
Mean	57.46		60.57		54.13	
Standard deviation	49.45		48.88		49.84	
R^2	.11		.12		.09	
Total (N)	(4,748)		(2,450)		(2,298)	

[a]The sum of total role losses occurring in (1969–1973).
[b]Indicators measured in 1973.
*Significant at .05 or lower level.

Our data do not provide evidence of a direct link between major-role loss and use of physician's services. The major-role losses were not significantly related to the likelihood of visiting a physician in either 1972 (table 4-10) or 1974 (table 10-11). A history of prior visits to a physician was a strong predictor of visits in later years.

The findings on the relationship between major-role losses and hospitalization are rather obscure. Although role loss was associated with hospitalization in 1972 among the total population, and among workers, this variable (it is surprising to observe), did not have a significant associa-

tion among retirees. Major-role losses were not significantly related to hospitalization in 1974 in the total population or in the retired or worker
subgroups. In fact, during this year, those who had major-role losses between 1969 and 1973 were less likely to be hospitalized. It may be that the
absence of significant others who could refer respondents to doctors or for
hospitalization contributed to this finding.

Our analysis thus far indicated that cumulative role losses do appear to
have some impact on health status, life satisfaction, and level of disability,
even when prior status in these areas is controlled. However, major role
losses do not have a significant effect on respondents' use of physicians' services and have only a slight influence on the likelihood of hospitalization.

We noted, in our analysis, some differences in the effects of major role
losses depending upon whether respondents were working or retired.
However, when major role losses were considered individually, retirement
appeared to have little influence on physical or psychological well-being, except in those groups that retired at somewhat earlier ages.

When the same controls are applied in the following chapter, we will examine the effects of retirement on health status in greater detail, observing
the effects of this event when prior health and psychological status are taken
into account.

References

1. Nye, F.I., and L.W. Hoffman "Husband-Wife Relationship," in
L.W. Hoffman and F.I. Nye, *Working Mothers* (New York: Jossey-Bass
Inc., 1974).

2. Hill, R. "Social Stresses on the Family," in Marvin Sussman, ed.,
Sourcebook of Marriage and the Family (Boston: Houghton-Mifflin Co.,
1968).

3. Lopata, H.Z., "The Social Involvement of American Widows,"
American Behavioral Scientist 14(1970):41–57.

4. Blau, Z., "Structural Constraints on Friendship in Old
Age,"*American Sociological Review* 26(1961):429–439.

5. Cavan, R., "The Couple in Old Age," in R. Cavan ed.. *Marriage
and the Family in the Modern World* (New York: Thomas Y. Cromwell
Co., 1969).

6. Berardo, F., "Survivorship and Social Isolation: The Case of the
Aged Widower," *The Family Coordinator* 19(1970):11–25.

7. Atchley, R., "Dimensions of Widowhood in Later Life," *The
Gerontologist* 15(1975):176–187.

8. Uhlenberg, P., and M.A. Myers, "Divorce and the Elderly," *The
Gerontologist* 21(1981):276–282.

9. Gove, W.R., "Sex, Marital Status and Psychiatric Treatment: A Research Note," *Social Forces* 58(1979):89–93.

10. Johnson, E.S., and B. Bursk, "Relationships Between the Elderly and Their Adult Children." *The Gerontologist* 17(1977):90–96.

11. Shanas, E., "Family and Household Characteristics of Older People in the United States," in F. Hansen, ed., *Age With a Future* (Copenhagen: Munksgaard, 1964).

12. Jacobson, D., "Rejection of the Retired Role: A Study of Female Industrial Workers in The Future," *Human Relations* 27(1974):477–492.

13. Streib, G., and C. Schneider, *Retirement in American Society* (New York: Cornell University Press, 1971).

14. Lopata, H.Z., "Widows as a Minority Group," *The Gerontologist* 11(1971):67–77.

15. Elwell, F., and A.D. Maltbie-Crannell, "The Impact of Role Loss Upon Coping Resources and Life Satisfaction of the Elderly," *Journal of Gerontology* 36(1981):223–232.

16. Thompson, G.B., "Work Versus Leisure Roles: An Investigation of Morale Among Employed and Retired Men," *Journal of Gerontology* 28(1973):339–344.

17. Nelson, L., and M. Winter, "Life Disruption, Independence, Satisfaction and the Consideration of Moving," *The Gerontologist* 15(1975):160–164.

18. Gubrium, J.J., "Marital Desolation and Evaluation of Everyday Life in Old Age," *Journal of Marriage and the Family* 36(1974):107–113.

19. Eckenrode, J., and S. Gore, "Successful Events and Social Supports: The Significance of Context," in B.H. Gottlieb, ed. *Social Networks and Social Support in Community Mental Health.* (Beverly Hills, Calif.: Sage Publications, Inc., 1981).

20. Foner, A., and S. Schwab, *Aging and Retirement* (Monterey, Calif.: Brooks/Cole Publishing Co., 1980).

21. Barfield, R.E., and J. Morgan, "Trends in Satisfaction with Retirement," *The Gerontologist* 18(1978):19–23.

22. Niemi, Timo "The Mortality of Male Old Age Pensioners Following Spouses' Deaths," *Scandinavian Journal of Social Medicine* 18(1979):115–117.

23. Rees, W., and S. Lutkins, "Mortality of Bereavement," *British Medical Journal* (1967), pp. 13–16.

24. Young, M., and P. Willmatt, *Family and Kinship in East London.* (London: Routledge and Kegan Paul, 1975).

25. Maddison, D., and A Viola, "The Health of Widows in the Year Following Bereavement," *Journal of Psychosomatic Research* 12(1968):297–306.

26. Heyman, O.K., and D.T. Gianturco, "Long-Term Adaptation by

the Elderly to Bereavement," *Journal of Gerontology* 28(1973):359–362.

27. Lowenthal, M.F., and D. Chiroboga, "Responses to Stress," in M.F. Lowenthal, M. Thurner, and D. Chiroboga, ed., *The Four Stages of Life* (San Francisco: Jossey-Bass, Inc., 1975).

28. Atchley, C., *The Social Forces in Later Life* (Belmont, Calif.: Wadsworth Publishing Co., 1980).

29. Kingston, E., "The Health of Very Early Retirees," *Aging and Work* (Winter 1981), pp. 11–22.

30. Andrisani, J., "Effects of Health Problems on Work Experience of Middle-Aged Men," *Industrial Gerontology* 4, no. 2 (1977):97–112.

31. Bixby, L.E., "Retirement Patterns in the U.S. Research and Policy Interaction," *Social Security Bulletin* (1976), pp. 3–19.

32. Parnes, H.S., and J. Jeyers, "Withdrawal from the Labor Force by Middle-Aged Men, 1966–1967," in G.M. Shattox, ed., *Employment of Middle-Aged Men* (Springfield, Ill.,: Charles C. Thompson, 1972).

33. Parnes, H.S., and G. Nestel, *Early Retirement in the Pre-Retirement Years, Volume 4.* (Washington, D.C.: U.S. Department of Labor, U.S. Government Printing Office, 1975).

34. Reno, V.P., "Why Men Stop Working at/or Before Age 65: Findings From the Survey of New Beneficiaries," *Social Security Bulletin* (1971), pp. 3–4.

35. Schwab, K. "Early Labor Force Withdrawal of Men: Participants and Non-Participants Aged 58–63," in *Almost 65. Baseline Data From the Retirement History,* (Washington, D.C.: Social Security Administration, U.S. Government Printing Office, 1976).

36. Sheppard, H.D., "Factors Associated with Early Withdrawal from the Labor Force," in S.L. Wolfbein, ed., *Men in Pre-Retirement Years.* (Philadelphia, Penn.: Temple University, Press, 1977).

37. Kimmel, D.C., K.S. Price, and J.W. Walker, "Retirement Choice and Retirement Satisfaction," *Journal of Gerontology* 33(1978):575–585.

38. Ward, R., *The Aging Experience* (New York: Harper and Row, Inc.,d 1979).

39. Riley, M., and A. Foner, *Aging and Society Volume 1: An Inventory of Research Finding* (New York: Russell Sage Foundation, 1968).

5 Health Effects of Retirement

Previous research on the nature of the relationship between retirement as a major role loss and health status has been reviewed in chapters 1 and 4. Briefly summarized, the findings from several cross-sectional and longitudinal studies do not lead us to draw strong conclusions on whether or not retirement will adversely affect health status.

However, a review of current research on life-change events and illness led us to hypothesize that a major-role loss, such as retirement, might contribute to a decline in health status. The role of retirement as an etiological or a stress-inducing factor has yet to be empirically explored in a prospective study.

In this chapter, we will begin by examining differentials in health status between working and retired persons. Next, we will test several of the models of the relationship between retirement and health status that were proposed in chapter 1. The use of panel data of the Longitudinal Retirement History Study will yield results that are pertinent to provide empirical answers for the following questions: (1) Does retirement concomitantly occur with many life-change events? (2) Does poor health determine the retirement decision? and (3) Does retirement adversely affect the health of the elderly when controlling for prior health status?

Analysis of Panel Data

In chapter 2 we observed that approximately 75 percent of the total population sampled retired over the entire six-year period studied. It should be noted at this point that the proportion of those who retired during each of the three periods of this study did vary. About 24 percent of the population of those who were working in 1969 retired during 1969–1971. Of those who were still working in 1971, about 41 percent retired during 1971–1973; of those who were working in 1973 about 53 percent retired during 1973–1975. The increasing percentages of retirees in each period no doubt reflects the advancing age of our panel.

In addressing the questions posed in the introduction to this chapter, it is necessary to keep in mind the varying proportions of those who entered retirement in each time period.

Concomitance of Retirement with Other Life-Change Events

Table 5-1 shows the correlation coefficients of retirement with other life-change events during the three study periods. Life-change events are categorized as major role losses, other life events, and declining health status.

The most obvious finding from this table is that retirement occurring in all three periods is most strongly associated with the category of other life-change events. In all three study periods, retirement is significantly associated with the other age-related events of living alone and experiencing a decline in economic status. Retirement is also significantly related to the event of marriage in the last study period. This is certainly a reflection of increased numbers of persons (mostly males in our sample) who at a more advanced age become widowed and subsequently remarry.

Table 5-1

Correlation Coefficients of Retirement with Other Life-Change Events in Three Periods: 1969-1971, 1971-1973, and 1973-1975

Life-Change Events in a Given Period [a]	Retirement Occurring in Three Periods [b]		
	RET1	RET2	RET3
Role Loss			
Widowhood	.062*	.040*	.076*
Divorce	−.005	−.023	.020
Separation	−.004	−.036*	.040*
Departure of children	.042*	.058*	.013
Other Life Events			
Marriage	.023	.024	.133*
Living alone	.065*	.058*	.065*
Decline of economic status	.127*	.154*	.208*
Poor health			
Self-assessed health	.136*	.136*	.090*
Dissatisfaction of health	.077*	.043*	.028
Disability levels	.218*	.194*	.032
(Total Number)	(5,386)	(3,914)[c]	(2,219)[d]

[a]The presence of an event is coded as 1, and otherwise as 0.

[b]The correlation of retirement in a given period (for example, retirement during 1969-1971, RET1) to a specific life event occurring in the same period as shown here.

[c]Retirees in 1971 were excluded.

[d]Retirees in 1969-1973 were excluded.

*Significant at .05 or lower level.

As found in chapter 4, retirement in this analysis does not occur concomitantly with other major role losses. However, retirement did have a consistent and significant relationship with widowhood, and it was also significantly related to the departure of the last child from the family during the earlier periods of our study. This latter finding probably reflects the age of the cohort at this time in the study.

There were a number of significant associations between retirement and poor health as measured by a decline in self-assessed health, an increase in dissatisfaction with life, and a rise in disability levels. While retirement was significantly associated with poor health in each of the first two periods of the study (1969–1971, 1971–1973), it was significantly related only to a decline in the area of self-assessed health in 1975. This may be because those who were most dissatisfied with their lives and who experienced severe disability retired at earlier ages.

In summary, our analysis of correlations seems to indicate that retirement is associated, to some extent, with a decline in health status, at least during the early periods of our study. However, the results of correlation analysis cannot provide answers to the question of whether retirement, per se, causes a decline in health. This issue will be examined later in this chapter.

Determinants of Retirement

Table 5–2 addresses the question of what factors determine the decision to retire. Three sets of factors are considered: race/sex, age cohort, and prior health status. Table 5–2 displays the results of a multiple-classification analysis of the probability of retiring in each of the three periods studied. As stated at the beginning of this chapter, probability of retirement is calculated based upon those who retired in each period but who were working in the prior study period. The table shows both unadjusted probabilities (P) and the probabilities (P') for each variable adjusted for all other variables included in this analysis.

Results in table 5–2 indicate that age is clearly the most significant predictor variable of the probability of retiring. The strong positive relationship found between age and retirement deserves in-depth commentary. In the first period of our study, age and retirement appear to be linearly related with the oldest age group most likely to retire ($P' = .57$). In the second and third study periods the relationship between age and retirement is curvilinear. In period two, those who were sixty-two years old in 1969, and who were between the ages of sixty-four and sixty-six years in the period 1971–1973, were most likely to retire. Likewise, in period three, those who were sixty years old in 1969 and who were between the ages of sixty-four and sixty-six years in the period 1973–1975 were most likely to retire. Clearly

Table 5-2
Multiple Classification Analysis of the Probability of Retirement in Three Periods (1969-1971, 1971-1973, and 1973-1975), by Demographic and Prior Health Status

Explanatory Factors	1969-1971		1971-1973		1973-1975	
	P	P'	P	P'	P	P'
Race/sex	(.08)[a]		(.03)		(.03)	
White male	.22	.22	.42	.41	.53	.53
White female	.22	.24	.35	.37	.50	.52
Nonwhite male	.31	.30	.42	.42	.53	.53
Nonwhite female	.34	.34	.34	.34	.49	.46
Age cohort in 1969	(.33*)		(.27*)		(.18*)	
58	.10	.10	.27	.27	.41	.41
59	.12	.12	.31	.31	.60	.59
60	.24	.24	.38	.38	.66	.65
61	.28	.28	.56	.56	.54	.54
62	.30	.30	.62	.62	.51	.51
63	.57	.57	.54	.54	.53	.53
Prior health status						
Self-assessed health	(.02)		(.06)		(.02)	
Poor	.28	.29	.40	.40	.50	.57
Good	.24	.24	.56	.53	.53	.53
Life satisfaction	(.04)		(.02)		(.04)	
Dissatisfied	.30	.29	.41	.41	.45	.49
Satisfied	.23	.23	.45	.44	.54	.54
Disability status			(.07)		(.08)	
Severe disability			.36	.25	.30	.32
Moderate disability			.54	.51	.60	.60
Minor disability			.49	.48	.59	.59
No disability			.39	.40	.52	.52
R^2	.12		.09		.04	
Grand mean	.24		.41		.53	
(Total N)	(5,386)		(3.914)[b]		(2,219)[c]	
(P = unadjusted proportion; P' = adjusted proportion)						

[a]Net effect (beta coefficient) of a categorized variable.
[b]Retirees in 1969-1971 were excluded.
[c]Retirees in 1969-1973 were excluded.
*The effect of a categorical variable on the probability of having retired is statistically significant at .05 or lower level.

the linear relationship between retirement and age observed in period one is only an artifact of the age of the cohort. In all three periods studied, retirement is most likely to occur around the age of sixty-five years.

The race-sex variable does not appear to be significantly related to the decision to retire. It is interesting to observe, however, that nonwhite females were more likely to retire during the first period of the study than other age-sex categories.

Health status had no significant impact on the decision to retire. There are two reasons to account for this: (1) the functionally disabled were excluded from our study sample at the outset, and (2) any variations in the retirement decision due to health are also attributed to the aging of the cohort. Thus, health factors do not appear to be significant when the effect of age is controlled. We should further observe that retirees in the second and third periods of this study were most likely to be the moderately or mildly disabled rather than the severely impaired. It is reasonable to assume that most of the severely disabled might involuntarily retire at earlier ages.

Effects of Retirement on Health Status

In the previous section, we observed that health status had a negligible influence on the decision to retire when age factor was taken into account. In order to examine the impact of retirement on health status, we performed path analysis. According to conventional path analysis, the correlation coefficient may be considered as the total independent effect of an independent variable on a dependent variable. The total effect consists of the direct effect and indirect effect. The direct effect is measured by a standardized partial-regression coefficient or path coefficient. The path coefficient, or beta weight, is standardized so that the comparison made between different variables will have meaning [1]. It denotes that a difference of one standard deviation on an independent variable will cause a certain corresponding variation on a dependent variable.

In figure 5–1, the values following the arrows express the direct effect of retirement and prior health status on the dependent variables of health status in 1973 and 1975. Health status is measured by three indicators: (1) self-assessed health, (2) life satisfaction, and (3) disability.

As shown in figure 5–1, retirement occurring in the first study period had a negligible effect on self-assessed health, life satisfaction, or disability measured in 1973 and 1975, when prior health status was controlled. This finding has further substantiated the fact the retirement does not cause maladaptation as manifested by ill health and dissatisfaction with life [2–5].

The importance of this result should not be underestimated. It should be stressed that no previous prospectively designed studies have examined the effects of retirement on health among a sample that was fundamentally healthy at the beginning of the study. Further, the prospective nature of this study design enabled us to follow the sample from the time of retirement over a period of six years; thus our findings are not subject to errors in recall or to memory bias. According to our results, prior health status pro-

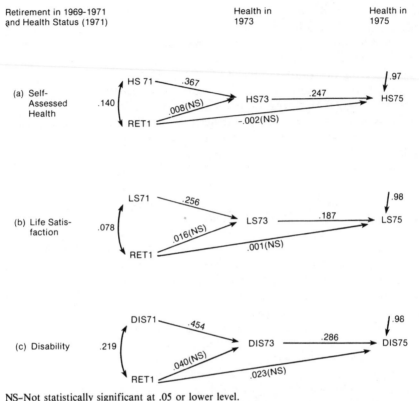

Retirement in 1969-1971   Health in   Health in
and Health Status (1971)   1973   1975

NS-Not statistically significant at .05 or lower level.

Figure 5-1. The Relationship between Retirement and Health Indicators, Controlling for Prior Health Status

vides the key to understanding future health among retirees. The act of retirement, in itself, does not exert a direct causal effect on health.

In order to reconfirm the results of path analysis, we performed cross tabulations of retirement for all three measures of health status, controlling for prior health. Results in table 5-3 demonstrate that, while there were appreciable differences in the total population in the numbers who perceived their health as getting worse or better, there was almost no difference in the self-perception of health status in 1973 and 1975 between persons who retired between 1969-1971 and those who continued to work. The same findings are apparent with regard to life satisfaction. Again, there were no differences between the working and retired.

Table 5-3 does show some differences between retirees and workers in the proportion of persons reporting functional limitations in 1973 and 1975. Retirees were somewhat more likely to be functionally disabled, even when

Table 5-3

The Effect of Retirement (1969–1971) on Self-Assessed Health in 1973 and 1975, Controlling for Prior Health Status

| Health and Retirement Status in 1971 | Persons Who Perceived Themselves as Having Worse Health Than Others of the Same Age | | | |
| | 1973 | | 1975 | |
	N	Percentage	N	Percentage
Worse health	216	56.5	172	49.7
Same/better health	448	9.5	626	14.2
Worse health				
Retired	97	58.4	76	50.7
Working	119	55.1	96	49.0
Same/better health				
Retired	100	9.7	128	13.9
Working	348	9.4	498	14.3

prior disability status was controlled. We may infer that there may be some link between retirement and subsequent report of functional limitations. However, the path analysis suggests that this link is weak. One explanation of this finding may be that the report of functional limitations among the retired may be used to psychologically justify retirement, since all other measures of health status do not indicate differences between retirees and workers. Another explanation may be that report of functional limitation is a more objective measure of health than self-assessed health or life satisfaction. Further research to gather information outside the scope of this study will be necessary to determine the validity of these alternative explanations.

Discussion

The two key findings of this chapter deserve reiteration because of their importance to the understanding of the retirement process. These findings are:

1. Age is the principal determinant of the decision to retire.
2. Retirement, studied prospectively, has no significant effect on health status (as measured by self-assessed health, life satisfaction, and disability status) when prior health status is controlled.

The finding of a strong effect on retirement implies the importance of chronological age to the retirement decision. Two methodological issues need to be addressed in future studies. First, the relative influence of age, period, and cohort on the retirement process should be studied using a large representative sample of preretirement population. In this context, period refers to the historical time at which retirement occurs, and cohort refers to the psychological commonalities shared by a group of people who pass through stages of the life cycle at the same time. Our data indicate that, of the three concepts, chronological age is of prime importance in determining the decision to retire. In all three periods of our study and in each age cohort, retirement occurred around the age of sixty-five years. However, our findings in this area are far from conclusive. In order to identify the confounding effects of age, cohort, and period on retirement, time-series-study design is imperative so that a longer time period (at least forty years) with a wider range of age cohorts may be considered. Such an investigation is beyond the scope of the present study. Our findings do suggest that this subject deserves more careful consideration in future research.

Our second finding, that retirement is not an etiological factor in ill health has significant implications for future research and the development of policy to facilitate adjustment to retirement. Sociological research has long hinted that retirement, rather than having a detrimental effect on health, may have no effect or may actually result in an improvement in health, since for many people who dislike their jobs retirement represents a new sense of freedom [6]. Nonetheless, to date there has been little empirical evidence that health status at the time of retirement, rather than the event of retirement, explains variations in health that have been observed between retirees and workers. The findings of one recent study indicating that coronary-heart disease is a risk factor in the decision to retire rather than the reverse, tends to support our findings [7].

From a policy perspective, our findings suggest that the encouragement of preventive practices in the preretirement years may be the best way to ensure the future health of retired persons. Moreover, the results imply that poor health cannot be attributed to retirement alone. Our results lead us to believe that retirement may occur concomitantly with a series of age-related life changes, including a decline in economic status, marriage, or more likely remarriage, and a change to living alone. This synergistic effect of retirement and other life events has been noted elsewhere in the literature [8, 9], but, until now, have not been empirically demonstrated. The impacts of life changes associated with retirement on health status will be explored in depth in chapter 7.

References

1. Duncan, O.D., "Path Analysis: Sociological Examples," *American Journal of Sociology* 72 (1966):1-16.

2. Atchley, R., *The Social Forces in Later Life* (Belmont, Calif.: Wadsworth Publishing Co., 1980).

3. Thompson, G.B., "Work Versus Leisure Roles: An Investigation of Morale Among Employed and Retired Men," *Journal of Gerontology* 28 (1973):339–344.

4. Streib, G., and C. Schneider, *Retirement in American Society* (Ithaca, New York: Cornell University Press, 1971).

5. Mutran, E., and D.C. Reitzes, "Retirement, Identity and Well-Being: Realignment of Role Relationships," *Journal of Gerontology* 36 (1981):733–740.

6. Fischer, P.H., *Growing Old in America* (New York: Oxford University Press, 1977).

7. Gonzales, E.R., "Retiring May Predispose to Fatal Heart Attack," *Journal of the American Medical Association* 243 (1980):13–14.

8. Portnoi, V.A., "The Natural History of Retirement," *Journal of the American Medical Association* 245 (1981):1752–1754.

9. Minkler, M., "Research on the Health Effects of Retirement: An Uncertain Legacy," *Journal of Health and Social Behavior* 22, no. 2 (1981): 117–130.

6

Social-Support
Networks in Later Life

In this chapter we will explore the availability of social-support networks in terms of children, siblings, other relatives, and friends, and the intensity of these relationships. As documented in earlier research, children are considered a major source of support for some elderly [1]; however, as Eckenrode and Gore [2] point out, there may be variations between the number of people who potentially could give support and the number who actually do.

Recent research indicates a possible link between life-change events, social support, health status, and service utilization. The discovery of a causal link among these variables for the elderly could have relevance for future policy in aging.

Clearly, the rising costs of providing geriatric social services through the formal service-delivery network have generated an intense interest in reaching a better understanding of the importance of informal-support network, as family and friends. In addition, findings concerning the relevance of social support may have importance for the understanding of the phenomenon of change and the significance of social networks at all stages in the family life-cycle.

The two objectives of this chapter are (1) to review previous research on the conceptualization of social support and its hypothesized relationship to health and use of health services, and (2) to examine the differentials and magnitude of social support in the Longitudinal Retirement History population and the relationship of social support to major role losses. Two entire chapters of this book (seven and eight) will present our findings on the relationship of social support to health and health-services utilization.

Related Research

Definitions of Social Support

Lin et al. [3] have defined social support as "support accessible to an individual through social ties to other individuals, groups and the larger community." The characteristics of social support have been outlined by Bowlby [4] in his attachment theory. This theory states that each person requires a set of relationships that provides:

Meaningful attachment to significant others;

Social integration in a network of common interest relationships;

An opportunity for the nurturing of others, especially of children;

Reassurance of individual worth gained through the performance of a valued social role;

A sense of reliable alliance with kin;

Access to guidance from a trustworthy and authoritative person in times of stress.

In summation, social support allows an individual to feel cared for and loved, provides a feeling of social worth, and allows him to see himself as part of a network of communication and mutual obligation [5].

A number of approaches may be taken to conceptualize social support. Longino and Lipman [6] outline two. One approach examines the *provision of support,* that is, the kinds of support given. Gore [2] has identified two principal types of support, instrumental in which task-oriented help is given, and expressive support in which emotional support is given. Another way to approach social support is to examine the *dynamics of the support system.* With this approach, interrelationships between the social, emotional, and economic dimensions of the support system are explored [8].

This could be considered a normative approach to social support. A more positivistic approach to social support is to describe it in terms of the social network [9]. This approach allows evaluation of support in terms of measureable characteristics.

Mitchell [10] describes the characteristics of social networks, dividing them into two categories using morphological and interaction criteria. Morphological characteristics refer to the relationship or patterning of the links in the network with respect to one another. These include reachability, density, and range. Reachability refers to the ability of the individual to contact others in his network and their ability to contact him. Range is the number of people with whom the individual is in direct contact, and density is the extent to which persons in the network interact with one another, or the ratio of actual links to potential ones.

Interaction criteria refer to the nature of the links themselves and include content, directedness, intensity, and frequency. Content is the meaning those in the network give their relationships. The relationship may be multiplex, having more than one meaning; for example, kinship obligation and economic assistance may both be present in a relationship. Directedness may be one-directional or reciprocal. Durability refers to the length of time a contact continues; this may be for a lifetime or only for a brief period. The intensity of the linkage is the degree to which individuals are prepared to honor obligations, or feel free to exercise the rights implied in their link to some other persons. Finally, frequency is the regularity of contact between the individual and network members. High frequency, however, does not necessarily imply high intensity in the relationship.

Social Support and Health

Shanas [1] has documented the availability of kin to provide support for the elderly. She reports that 91 percent of parents sixty-five years and over receive some help from their children in the form of gifts, help during sickness, financial aid, or general advice.

A review of the literature relating social support to health illustrates the many ways that support has been measured in health-related research. Type of help received reflects the content and intensity of the network [11]. Availability of network members could take into account reachability, density, and range of the network [12, 13]. Also, the rate of interaction with family and friends may be measured [3, 14, 15]. This takes into consideration frequency, density, and range of the individual's social network. In some cases, social support is measured by simply looking at living arrangements, [16, 17] or the presence and nature of marital relationships [1, 18, 19–21].

There have been numerous studies that demonstrate that social support does have some impact on health status and health-related behavior [12, 14, 22, 23, 24]. For example, Lin et al. [3] employed a twenty-six item scale, which tapped the extent to which instrumental and expressive support was adequate or inadequate, to demonstrate that the absence of social support was a significant factor in the epidemiology of depression among diverse age groups. Among the oldest group in this study, marital status and history of previous illness also contributed to the explained variance in depression.

Similarly, Wan and Weissert [24] found that the presence of social-support networks had a positive effect on the health status of a group of elderly involved in a day-care and homemaker-service experiment. In this study, a scale of six items that indicated the presence or absence of social contact with spouse, children, siblings, grandchildren, other relatives, and friends was constructed. It was found that availability of siblings, other relatives, and friends was associated with high levels of physical and mental functioning. Further, living with others and having children was inversely related to the likelihood of institutionalization.

Life Change, Social Support, and Health

A second group of studies considered social support as having a mediating or buffering effect on stress produced by life changes, and ill health [7, 25–

30]. (See appendix for a complete summary of empirical findings on this subject.) These studies, in general, have not offered strong evidence for the buffering effect of social support against stress produced by life change. The studies of Fuller and Larson [3] and Peznecker and McNeil [28] produced no evidence that social support acted as a buffer against life change.

On the other hand, the studies of Palmore [27], Nuckolls et al. [26], Lowenthal and Haven [25], and Niemi [21] do provide some evidence for the mediating role of social support. For example, Palmore found that the impacts of widowhood, retirement, and departure of the children from the family on health were ameliorated by the presence of high social resources. Social resources were defined in terms of income, education, and density of the social network.

Also, specific to the experience of the aged are the findings of Gore's [7] study of involuntary job loss. Comparing two groups of recently unemployed males, one with low and the other with high social support, Gore found that, while no differences between the two groups existed in reemployment rates or in the amount of economic deprivation experienced, the group with higher social support manifested less self-blame and depression and had fewer physiological symptoms of illness. Her findings pertain to the situation of the involuntary retired male and suggest the buffering effect of support. The value of support for the elderly in mitigating other changes involving loss is also documented. Lowenthal and Haven [25] report that, among their elderly sample, those who decreased their social interaction and who did not have a confidante were more often depressed than those with a confidante or increased interaction. In the area of bereavement, the studies of Parker and Burch both reveal an inverse relationship between contact with others and risk of mental illness [5].

Social Support and Utilization

Several studies have related social support to forms of service utilization other than institutionalization [14, 17, 18]. Murdock and Swartz [17] report that awareness of service agencies and use of agency services was higher among those elderly living in extended family settings.

A study that should shed some light on the relationship between life change, social support and health is currently underway under the direction of Steven Gortmaker of the Harvard School of Public Health. Subjects in this study are women who have at least one dependent child under twenty-five. In this study, previous history of life change is recorded and subjects are asked to keep diaries of the stress they experience daily. Social support is measured by frequency of contact with relatives, number of potential helpers in problem situations, and the degree of social participation or integration experienced. Utilization of medical services is indicated by physicians' ratings of the degree to which the complaint merits medical treatment. This study builds upon the work of Robert J. Haggarty who found that stress did increase use of physician's services. The results of the Gortmaker study and our prospective study among an elderly population should enhance our knowledge of the functions of social support in service utilization.

Evaluation of previous research on the effects of social support is hampered by lack of a clear, consistent definition of support. In addition, many previous studies that have sought to discern the interrelationships between life change, social support, and illness are retrospective. At this time, it is difficult to reach a definite conclusion on the relationship between social support and health, or to discern the importance of social support as a buffer against life changes.

Our own research clarifies the relationship between social support and health status through the use of panel data. Further, the use of multiple indicators of social support enhances the comparability of our study with previous research. In the current study, the variable social support is measured by the following indicators: (1) living arrangements, (2) marital status, and (3) the breadth and intensity of interaction in the social network.

Marital status includes the categories of married, widowed, divorced, separated, or single. Living arrangements is a dichotomized variable defined as living alone or with others. The social network is measured in terms of the presence or absence of children, siblings, relatives, and friends. From this description of the network, a weighted measure of the importance of the foregoing relationships is derived based upon frequency of interaction.

Our findings concerning the magnitude of social networks and their multiplicity are presented in the following sections.

Analysis

Social Networks: Trends and Differentials

Table 6–1 displays trends in the social-support-network scores between the years 1971 and 1975 by race and sex while controlling for marital status and living arrangements. These two latter factors may also affect the level of social support. The social-support-network score is a composite index indicating the presence or absence of contacts with children, siblings, other relatives, and friends and the frequency of interaction, scored as daily (4), weekly (3), monthly (2), less than monthly (1), and no interaction (0). The social support network score ranges from 0 for no contact to 16 for daily contacts with each of the four types of social resources mentioned. The derivation of the social support score can be summarized as follows:

$$\sum_{i=1}^{4} \quad \begin{array}{l} \text{Presence or absence of a} \\ \text{special type of social} \\ \text{support } (1,0) \end{array} \quad \times \quad \begin{array}{l} \text{Intensity of} \\ \text{interaction} \\ (0\text{--}4) \end{array}$$

Table 6–1 shows that the average composite social-network score was 8.7 in 1971. The original composition of our sample, which included married and unmarried males and which included married females in 1969, makes comparisons between the sexes risky. Our data indicate that nonwhite females had the highest social network score (8.9). This was slightly higher than the score for white females (8.4). White males, on the other hand, had higher network scores (8.8) than nonwhite males (8.4). That the scores for females are higher than the scores for males is consistent with previous findings [6].

The differences in composite social-support scores between racial groups within marital status categories raises important questions. To what degree does the concept of the family unit differ between racial groups and consequently alter participation in the social network? For instance, does a greater acceptance of one-parent households among nonwhites offer greater opportunities for developing support networks outside the conjugal unit? Also, to what degree do differences in the availability of social supports due to differences in family size and so forth affect the amount of social support available?

When we look at differences in social-network scores among races, controlling for marital status, it is apparent that married persons had the highest social-support score (9.0) and single persons had the lowest (7.0). While we note an overall pattern that revealed high social-network scores for nonwhite females, this pattern is changed somewhat within marital-status categories. It is interesting to note that, among the widowed and the single, white females have a higher score (9.3) than nonwhite females (8.8); however, among the married, separated, and divorced, nonwhite females have higher scores.

Among males, nonwhites who were widowed, divorced, separated, or single have higher interaction scores than whites. Married white males, however, score higher (9.0) than nonwhite males (8.4).

Social support scores also vary by living arrangement. In general, persons living with others have higher social-support scores (8.9) than persons living alone (8.2), a finding that has previously been demonstrated. Among those living alone, females have a higher level of social support than males, while among those living with others, white males have more support. It is interesting to observe that level-of-social-support networks alters drastically for white males depending upon living arrangement. White males living with others have comparably high levels of support (8.9), and white males

Table 6-1
Average Social-Support Network Scores in 1971 and 1975 for Four Subgroups, by Marital Status and Living Arrangement

Characteristics	Total	White Males	White Females	Nonwhite Males	Nonwhite Females
1971					
Total (*N* = 5,386)	8.7	8.8	8.5	8.4	8.9
Marital status					
Married	9.0	9.0	8.6	8.4	10.7
Widowed	8.7	8.6	9.3	8.7	8.8
Divorced	8.1	7.5	7.3	8.4	8.4
Separated	8.1	7.6	7.5	8.5	9.3
Single	7.0	6.3	9.1	7.2	8.4
Living arrangement					
Living alone	8.2	7.8	8.6	8.4	9.3
Living with others	8.9	8.9	8.0	8.4	8.5
1975					
Total (*N* = 4,748)	7.7	7.9	7.4	7.5	6.9
Marital status					
Married	8.0	8.0	7.6	8.0	8.1
Widowed	7.8	8.0	7.0	7.9	6.7
Divorced	7.3	6.7	7.6	7.7	7.4
Separated	6.9	7.0	6.1	7.5	6.6
Single	5.8	5.7	5.8	5.7	6.4
Living arrangement					
Living alone	7.6	7.7	7.3	7.6	7.2
Living with others	7.8	7.9	7.4	7.2	6.6

living alone have comparably low levels (7.8). The difference probably reflects the influence of the spouse in making social contacts and in establishing relationships. This also explains the higher level of support among married white males.

Comparisons of our sample's social-support scores in 1971 with their scores in 1975 show an overall decline in the level of social support. Composite scores for the total sample dropped from 8.7 in 1971 to 7.7 in 1975. It has been proposed theoretically [31] and documented empirically that some decline in either breadth or intensity of interaction in the social network occurs with advancing age. Our data support this conclusion. Futhermore, nonwhite females appear to experience the decline in support most severely (scores of 8.9 in 1971 to 6.9 in 1975). Changes occurring between 1971 and 1975 in the Composite Index Scores of Social Support are displayed in figure 6-1.

While, in 1975, the pattern of support scores remained the same, with married persons having the highest level of support and single persons the

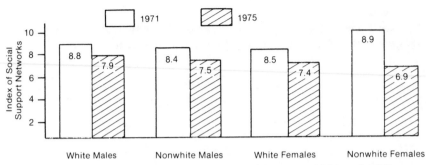

Figure 6-1. Composite Index of Social Support, 1971 and 1975

lowest, there were some differences within marital status categories in 1975 as compared to 1971. Although all racial and sex categories show diminished social support, it is noteworthy that the support of single white females declines drastically (9.1 in 1971 to 5.8 in 1975). Also, differences between white and nonwhite males are much less in this period.

Looking at living arrangements, those living with others still have higher levels of support in 1975, but differences in support on the basis of living arrangement are less. Surprisingly, both nonwhite males and females living with others have lower support scores (7.2 and 6.6) than those living alone (7.6 and 7.2).

Apparently, the nonwhite females who are living with others do not receive the social support that is often presumed to exist in this living arrangement.

Having examined differentials in the total social-support scores of the population studied in 1971 and 1975, we will now analyze the various sources of support by living arrangement and marital status. Tables 6-2 and 6-3 report the proportions of people with a specific type of social-support network in 1971 and in 1975.

Those receiving social support from children in 1971 were most likely to be nonwhite males living alone (57.4 percent), white males living with others (82.6 percent), married males (74.5 percent white and 75.8 percent nonwhite), and unmarried nonwhite males (53 percent). Clearly, in our study, males appear to receive more support from children than do females. However, again, this may be due to the fact that our sample excluded married females in 1969 and that many of the females included had never been married.

In 1971 our sample received proportionately more support from siblings, other relatives, and friends than from children. People most likely to have siblings in their social-support network were white males living alone (78.4 percent) or with others (89.8 percent), married, nonwhite females (100.0 percent) and nonmarried white males (79.8 percent). Females, both

Table 6-2
Proportions of Those with Specific Types of Social-Support Networks in 1971, by Social and Demographic Characteristics

| Characteristics | Type of Social-Support Network | | | |
	Child	Siblings	Other Relatives	Friends
Living alone				
White males	48.4	78.4	72.7	86.2
White females	47.9	71.4	95.7	89.8
Nonwhite males	57.4	76.0	37.4	91.0
Nonwhite females	47.4	76.3	94.2	89.5
Living with others				
White males	82.6	89.8	61.1	89.2
White females	51.3	86.3	67.5	86.3
Nonwhite males	47.2	78.5	68.9	87.8
Nonwhite females	49.2	81.4	66.3	91.5
Married				
White males	74.5	90.2	60.9	89.3
White females	52.8	86.6	67.2	85.5
Nonwhite males	75.8	93.9	63.6	90.9
Nonwhite females	66.7	100.0	100.0	100.0
Not married				
White males	43.6	79.8	59.8	86.5
White females	42.5	75.3	64.4	91.8
Nonwhite males	53.0	76.4	63.6	89.8
Nonwhite females	47.3	77.5	69.0	89.1

married and not married and females living alone, were more likely to include "other relatives" in their support networks. Nonwhites were generally more likely to include friends. However, it should be noted that among those not married, white females were most likely to report having friends in their social networks.

Since nonwhite females reported relatively high composite network scores in 1971, it is worthwhile to examine their network in more detail. Married nonwhite females appear to have a wider range of social support that includes siblings, other relatives, and friends.

In 1975, as shown in table 6-3, the pattern of support received changes. When respondents were younger (in 1971) a greater proportion of support was received from persons who, it may be assumed, were peers (siblings, relatives, and friends). In 1975, there was an increase in the proportion of respondents mentioning children in their support network. In 1975, a greater proportion of those living with others also reported support from siblings. Almost all categories considered also were more likely to include relatives in their social network, while the proportion of those including friends declined. This decline is particularly substantial for nonwhite

Table 6-3
Proportions of Those with Specific Types of Social-Support Networks in 1975, by Social and Demographic Characteristics

Characteristics	Type of Social-Support Network			
	Child	Siblings	Other Relatives	Friends
Living alone				
White males	65.4	70.6	93.8	77.2
White females	64.1	60.9	93.8	75.0
Nonwhite males	61.1	67.0	93.9	80.8
Nonwhite females	46.8	67.7	93.5	72.6
Living with others				
White males	78.5	97.4	97.4	78.2
White females	77.7	95.5	95.5	76.6
Nonwhite males	72.1	97.4	97.4	77.4
Nonwhite females	72.9	94.9	94.9	55.9
Married				
White males	82.0	79.1	97.6	78.9
White females	69.6	77.9	95.8	75.4
Nonwhite males	85.7	79.4	99.2	80.2
Nonwhite females	60.0	80.0	100.0	60.0
Not married				
White males	62.0	71.2	94.4	75.1
White females	52.7	65.6	93.5	78.4
Nonwhite males	56.5	67.7	94.9	79.2
Nonwhite females	50.5	69.4	93.7	64.9

females. Analysis of our tables thus far allows us to draw some conclusions on trends in the receipt of social support.

Combining our information from the composite indexes (table 6-1) with the data on multiplicity of network connections (tables 6-2, 6-3), we may conclude that the breadth of the social network increases with advancing age; however, the intensity of relationships appears to decline. This would account for the decline in the composite social-support score between 1971 and 1975 even though the multiplicity of sources of social support increases. It may be that, as one ages, a diversity of supports are needed. Support may change in nature from primarily one providing companionship to one providing other kinds of assistance—such as help with house maintenance or financial difficulties.

Major Role Losses and Social Support

Analysis of table 6-4 reveals that major role losses do not appear to be strongly associated with changes in the social-support network. In 1971,

Table 6-4
The Relationship of the Social-Support Network Score to
Role-Loss Variables

Role Losses in a Given Period	1971	1975
	r	r
Retirement	− .008 (NS)	− .001 (NS)
Widowhood	.017 (NS)	.027*
Divorce	− .001 (NS)	− .011 (NS)
Separation	− .008 (NS)	− .022 (NS)
Departure of Children	− .041*	.017 (NS)
Weighted Role-Loss Variable	− .025*	.015 (NS)

NS = Not statistically significant.
*Significant at .05 or lower level.

only departure of children was related to a change in the social-support net-work. As children depart from the home, social-support scores decline. In 1975, this relationship was not significant, perhaps due to fewer people experiencing this event at more advanced ages. It should be observed that the effect of departure of the children changes from reducing social support in 1971 to increasing it in 1975. It is possible that, at more advanced ages, the number of persons who have experienced this event provides a pool of support.

In 1975, the only role loss that had a significant effect on the social-support score was widowhood. Instead of reducing the social-support score, this event tended to increase it. This finding would seem to refute Eckhardt and Gore's vulnerability hypothesis which postulates that major roles constitute the foundation of the social-support network and that the loss of these roles reduces the social network [2].

This finding, however, is consistent with Blau's hypothesis that the number of persons experiencing a major-role loss within a cohort affects the amount of support received [32]. In 1975, there are more widowed in the population of our sample cohort, due to advancing age. This may account for a significant increase in the composite social-support score in 1975. It is especially interesting that retirement as a major role loss had no significant effect in 1971 and in 1975 on the composite social-support score.

In general, two conclusions may be reached from the findings of this chapter. First, everyone in our sample, regardless of race, sex, marital status, or living arrangement, appears to have some form of social support. This is not surprising given that the persons studied were all in good health in 1969 and had worked. We would expect that this population would have ties to family and be integrated, at least to some extent, into their communities. Our findings do imply that the stereotype of the isolated elderly person does not fit a sample of relatively healthy older people. Second, our findings tend to refute the notion that retirement as a major role loss has an impact on social support. To probe whether friendships associated with working life are maintained after retirement, or whether new friendships or nonwork-related friendships are developed, is beyond the scope of our study, but clearly deserves investigation in future research.

References

1. Shanas, E., "The Family as a Social Support System in Old Age," *The Gerontologist* 19 (1979):169–174.

2. Eckenrode, J., and S. Gore, "Stressful Events and Social Supports: The Significance of Context," in B.H. Gottlieb, ed., *Social Networks and Social Support in Community Mental Health* (Beverly Hills, Calif.: Sage Publications, 1981).

3. Lin, N., et al., "Social Support, Stressful Life Events, and Illness: A Model and an Empirical Test," *Journal of Health and Social Behavior* 20 (1979):108–119.

4. Caplan, G., *Support Systems and Community Mental Health: Lectures on Concept Development* (New York: Behavioral Publications, 1974).

5. Cobb, S., "Social Support as a Moderator of Life Stress," *Psychosomatic Medicine* 38 (1976):300–312.

6. Longino, D.F., and A. Lipman, "Married and Spouseless Men and Women in Planned Retirement Communities: Support Network Differentials," Paper presented at the Thirty-second Annual Meeting of the Gerontological Society in Washington, D.C., 1979.

7. Gore, S., "The Effect of Social Support in Moderating the Health Consequences of Unemployment," *Journal of Health and Social Behavior* 19 (1978):157–165.

8. Lopata, H.Z., "Contributions of the Extended Families to the Social Support Systems of Metropolitan Area Widows: Limtations of the Modified Kin Network," *Journal of Marriage and Family* 40 (1978):358–364.

9. Walker, K.N., et al., "Social Support Networks and the Crisis of Bereavement," *Social Science and Medicine* 11 (1977):35–41.

10. Mitchell, J.C., ed., *Social Networks and Urban Situations* (Manchester, Manchester University Press, 1969).

11. Croog, S.H., et al., "Help Patterns: The Roles of Kin Network, Non-Family Resources, and Institutions," *Journal of Marriage and the Family* 2 (1972):32–41.

12. Finlayson, A., "Social Networks as Coping Resources," *Social Science and Medicine* 10 (1976):47–103.

13. Horwitz, A., "Family, Kin, and Friend Networks in Psychiatric Help-Seeking," *Social Science and Medicine* 12 (1978):297–304.

14. Langlie, J.K., "Social Networks, Health Beliefs and Preventive Health Behavior," *Journal of Health and Social Behavior* 18 (1977):244–260.

15. Holzman, J.M., et al., "Health and Early Retirement Decisions," *Journal of the American Geriatric Society* 28 (1980):23–28.

16. Brody, S.J.; W. Poulshock; and C.F. Masciocchi, "The Family Caring Unit: A Major Consideration in the Long-Term Support System," *The Gerontologist* 18 (1978):556–561.

17. Murdock, S.H., and D.F. Schwartz, "Family Structure and the Use of Agency Services: An Examination of Patterns Among Elderly Native Americans," *The Gerontologist* 18 (1978):475–481.

18. Pratt, L., "Conjugal Organization and Health," *Journal of Marriage and the Family* 34 (1972):85–94.

19. Barney, J.L., "The Prerogative of Choice in Long-Term Care," *The Gerontologist* 17 (1977):309–314.

20. Niemi, T., "The Mortality of Male Old-Age Pensioners Following Spouses' Death," *Scandinavian Journal of Social Medicine* 7 (1979):115–117.

21. Niemi, T., "Effect of Loneliness on Mortality After Retirement," *Scandinavian Journal of Social Medicine* 7 (1979):63–65.

22. Slesinger, D.P., "The Utilization of Preventive Medical Services by Urban Black Mothers," in David Mechanic, ed., *The Growth of Bureaucratic Medicine* (New York: John Wiley and Sons, Inc., 1976).

23. Smith, R.T., "Rehabilitation of the Disabled: The Role of Social Networks in the Recovery Process," *International Rehabilitative Medicine* 1 (1979):63–72.

24. Wan, T.T.H., and W. Weissert, "Social Support Networks, Patient Status and Institutionalization," *Research on Aging* 3, no. 2 (1981): 240–256.

25. Lowenthal, M.F., and C. Haven, "Interaction and Adaptation: Intimacy as a Critical Valuable," *American Sociological Review* 33 (1968): 20–30.

26. Nuckolls, K.B., et al., "Psychosocial Assets, Life Crisis and the Prognosis of Pregnancy," *American Journal of Epidemiology* 95 (1972): 431–441.

27. Palmore, E., et al., "Stress and Adaptation in Later Life," *Journal of Gerontology* 34 (1979):841–851.

28. Pesznecker, B.C., and J. McNeil, "Relationtionship Among Health Habits, Social Assets, Psychological Well-Being, Life Change, and Alterations in Health Status," *Nursing Research* 24 (1975):442–447.

29. Eaton, W.W., "Life Events, Social Supports, and Psychiatric Symptoms," *Journal of Health and Social Behavior* 19 (1978):230–234.

30. Fuller, S.S., and S.B. Larson, "Life Events, Emotional Support, and Health of Older People," *Research in Nursing and Health* 3 (1980): 81–89.

31. Cumming, E., and W.E. Henry, *Growing Old: The Process of Disengagement* (New York: Basic Books, 1961).

32. Blau, Z., "Structural Constraints on Friendship in Old Age," *American Sociological Review* 26 (1961):429–439.

7

Gerontological Health and Social-Support Networks

Previous research has documented an inverse relationship between stressful life events and health [1-6]. These studies have primarily been based on retrospective study designs. Using this approach, identification of life-change events is often accomplished by asking individuals to recall past events, and this may cause errors through selective memory, denial of certan events, and possible underreporting [7]. The use of the prospective approach in studying actual life-change experiences will prove more valid and predictive of the future state of well-being.

In this chapter, we will examine the relationship between various health-status indicators and life events occurring at or near retirement age. The underlying theoretical framework used in this study is that life stress is induced by many change events in later life and that these events may adversely affect an older person's adjustment to life situations. Thus, we postulated that the more frequent the changes or deteriorations one has experienced, the lower the level of health or well-being reported and the greater the use of health services observed in retirement age. Furthermore, the effect of stressful life events on health and health care can be mediated by an intervening factor, social support. In order to tease out the causal chains or etiological sources of the decline in health, we performed multivariate analysis of four waves of panel data obtained from the Longitudinal Retirement History Study.

Related Research

There are often several life events occurring at or near retirement age. For instance, *decline of economic well-being* occurs at retirement: most older people experience a loss of income. Moreover, after retirement, a fixed income can mean a continuing deterioration in relative position within the income structure [8]. Sixty-nine percent of the retired men say their income is much smaller now than it was before retirement; another 24 percent say it is a little smaller. The longer a person lives after retirement, the lower his income status is likely to become as compared to the income of those still working.

Change in living arrangement may result from the departure of children or loss of spouse, leaving the individual living alone. Isolation which develops relatively late in life is quite stressful. It increases vulnerability to illness, accidents, malnutrition, and loneliness [9]. Katz et al. [10] employed type-of-living-arrangement as an explanatory factor in a study evaluating the effects of home care, and found significant differences between those who lived with others and those who lived alone, in terms of function, injury, mortality, and in use of services.

Changes in marital status, such as widowhood and divorce, were associated with lower reported well-being [11, 12]. Change in marital status through divorce or widowhood may precipitate changes in other areas such as living arrangement, place of residence, and income. Increasing dependency was found the number one cause of low morale among older people [13]. Apparently, the negative attitudes toward financial or physical dependency and the strong positive valuation of independence combine to undermine the general well-being of the dependent older person.

Occupational change is less likely to occur among the older than the younger workers [8]. However, if this change occurs in old age, it involves more emotional distresses, loss of working relationship, loss of income, and so forth, than in younger people.

Retirement. The retirement process, which is so often the portal through which the adaptation for role loss starts, can easily become the precipitating agent for mental and physical disorders. This statement remains speculative if no systematic research, using prospective study designs, validates this assumption. Previous research seems to indicate that retirement as a life-change event is not as stressful as had been expected [14, 15, 16]. Women appear to be more negatively affected by retirement than are men [14, 17]. Conditions surrounding retirement such as state of health and level of income are more important in determining morale and attitude after retirement than is actual loss of work role [15, 18]. Furthermore, the emotional impact of retirement is based on the cumulative effect of many factors such as the life-change events cited above.

The clustering of these life-change events may be considered as a necessary but not sufficient cause of illness and may account, in part, for the time of onset of disease [5].

More specifically, the clusters of life-change events are related to the onset of diseases as tuberculosis, glaucoma, inguinal hernia, rheumatoid arthritis, myocardial infarction, sudden cardiac death, duodenal ulcer, schizophrenia, depression, and so forth. The interpretation of the pathogenesis of life stress can be found in much of the psychosomatic-medicine literature. For instance, according to Cassel [19], social factors may increase the risk of ill health by increasing the general susceptability to disease. Thus, it would be useful to identify social situations related to poor health.

In testing the proposition that the onset of diseases occurs in a framework of mounting social stress, Rahe et al. [4] compared twenty employees in a tuberculosis sanatorium who contracted tuberculosis with twenty employees who were exposed to the same risk but did not contract the disease. Employees who became ill were characterized by a significant clustering of changes in social status. They also found significant clusterings of social stress in the previous two years for groups of patients with cardiac disease, skin disease, and inguinal hernia, and females experiencing pregnancy.

To further test this hypothesis, Holmes and Rahe [5] developed the Social Readjustment Rating Scale. They defined social readjustment as both intensity and length of time necessary to adapt to a life event regardless of its desirability. A sample of 394 subjects rated forty-three life events from 0 to 1,000 points. Marriage was given an arbitrary value of 500. From these scores a 100 point rating scale was devised with values from 11, for a minor violation of the law, to 100, for death of a spouse. To utilize the Social Readjustment Scale, a subject is asked to indicate all the events that have occurred within the previous two years. The points for each event are totaled for a score. When the score is high, the individual is considered at a high risk of illness. Holmes found 80 percent of those subjects who scored over 300 developed serious illness such as heart attack or pathological depression.

Several studies [20, 21, 22] have replicated the scale and revealed a remarkable consensus in the scaling of events. Moreover, there were high correlations between minority and white groups, as there were in studies comparing Americans to Japanese, West Europeans, and Mexican-Americans. Paykel et al. [23] found a high similarity between British and American scaling of events. Similarly, Wyler, Masuda, and Holmes [6] discovered a positive relationship between the amount of life change and the seriousness of illness. They used the scale with a sample of 332. The Seriousness of Illness Scale was used to measure illness. They stated that "life events assume etiological significance by evoking attempts at adaptation which are often accompanied by psychophysiologic reactions."

In examining life change and health in a sample of 536, Pesznecker and McNeil [3] found that life-change units were also positively related to illness. In addition, a high life-change score was the strongest predictor of ill health when compared to other variables, including health habits, psychological well-being, social support, and demographic variables.

A correlation between increased life-change and mental status was disclosed by Myers et al. [2]. In a sample of 720, increased life events were related to a worsening of mental symptomology. This finding was confirmed by Markusk and Favero [24] with a sample of 2,129. Life-event scores were related to depressed mood and psychophysiological symptoms.

Some studies have linked life-event scores to specific diseases. Theorell [25] scrutinized life events and early myocardial infarction. He found life-change buildups, especially problems with job or family, during the six months preceding onset of disease.

While stressful life events appear to be of etiological significance to illness, they do not necessarily affect everyone to the same extent. This suggests the possible influence of other variables on the etiological chain between life stress and illness. Rahe [26] suggests intervening steps between the occurrence of the event and the illness symptoms. First, participants tend to perceive events through individual fields of personal experience, some registering lower life-event scores, some higher for similar experiences. He feels that the values decrease with time; then, the individual's psychological defenses, physiological reaction, and coping devices (such as the ability to relax) may come into play.

Cobb [27] presents a different approach, originally offered by French and Kahn in 1962. This model has three levels of personal and environmental characteristics and the nature of the event:

Personal variables	psychological defenses
	psychological needs
	genetic predisposition
	past experience
	attitude toward illness
	illness behavior
Stress from event	role ambiguity
	future ambiguity
	work load
	cathected objects
	responsibility
Social factors	current life situation
	social support
	attitude of peers

Recent social epidemiological studies show that social support or social networks may either reduce the likelihood of illness as a predisposing factor, or serve as a buffer against the stress from life events [28]. Social support serves as a coping mechanism by (1) eliminating or modifying conditions that give rise to problems, (2) controlling the meaning of the experience in a manner that neutralizes the problematic character of the event, and (3) keeping the emotional consequences of problems within manageable bounds.

Lin et al. [28] theorized that strong social support would negate the effects of stressful life events. In the study of 550 Chinese-Americans, Lin and his associates found social support did mediate these effects. Subjects with high life-event scores and low social support had greater symptoms than did those with similar life-event scores and higher social support.

Cobb [29] defined social support as information leading the individual to believe that he is cared for and loved, esteemed and valued, and belonging to a network of mutual obligation. He reviews studies by Nuckolls et al. [30] who found excessive delivery complications among army wives with high life change and low social support. Brown et al. found that women who lacked a confidante were ten times more likely to become depressed than were women with a confidante. Cobb concluded that there is "hard evidence that adequate social support can protect people in crisis from a wide variety of pathological states." [27]

Research supporting this hypothesis includes Gore [31], who discovered lower levels of health symptoms among well-supported, unemployed men, and Lowenthal and Haven [32], who reported a relationship between depression and the lack of a confidante. Gore conducted a longitudinal study of the physical and mental consequences of unemployment among 174 workers. Social support modified the severity of both psychological and health responses to unemployment in her sample. Lowenthal and Haven interviewed 280 aged community residents on social roles and interaction. They deduced that individuals with a confidante could withstand the loss of social role without loss of morale.

Miller et al. [33] compared 172 people (with nine specific symptoms) who were consulters of physician's services to 172 nonconsulters. They characterized the consulters as individuals with high life-change events and few close friends.

DeAraujo et al. [34] studied the effects of life change and social support on the dosage of steroid required to treat thirty-six asthma patients. They utilized the life-events scale and a three-part Berle index which concerns demographic factors, medical history, questions on family and interpersonal relationships, and a physician's evaluation. Patients with low psychosocial assets and high life change required significantly higher doses of steroid compared to those with low assets and low life change. Patients with low psychosocial assets and high life change were continually incapacitated and needed constant medical care.

Longitudinal data on the life events, psychiatric symptoms, and social support of 720 subjects were analyzed by Eaton [35]. Life events had the strongest effect on subjects living alone and not married. Married subjects and those living with others suffered fewer symptoms from stressful life events. Thus, research to date reports that stress induced from life-change events may be mediated by social support.

Analysis of Panel Data

Researchers on life stress have developed a variety of scales, including weighted and unweighted indexes. The weighted index was developed in terms of the relative importance of life events affecting the life circumstance, while the unweighted index was the sum of the total events experienced by an individual during a specific period. In the study of life events experienced in three periods (1969–1971; 1971–1973; 1973–1975), we constructed a weighted index of stressful life events based upon the Holmes and Rahe's scoring as follows [5]:

Life-Change Events in Two Years	Scores
Retirement	45
Marriage	50
Widowhood	100
Divorce	73
Separation	65
Departure of children	29
Increased financial dependency	38
Change in living arrangement	25

The sum of the above eight-item scores constitutes a stress index for each study period. (The index of stressful life events does not include health-related items, since the SLE is considered a causal or etiological factor of poor health.) A combination of three stress scores (1969–1971, 1971–1973, and 1973–1975) represents the overall stress experienced by the elderly person from 1969–1975.

In order to determine the relationship of gerontological health to life events and social-support networks, a path analytic model is formulated to include health status and use of physician services as endogenous (dependent) variables, and life events, social-support networks, and prior health and utilization behavior as exogenous variables (see figure 7-1). Prior status, life events experienced in 1969–1971, and social support networks are considered correlates and are assumed to affect health and the use of physician services causally.

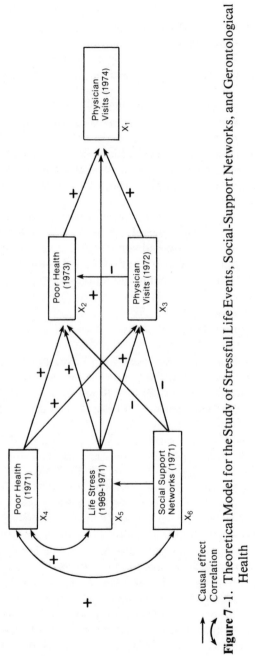

Figure 7–1. Theoretical Model for the Study of Stressful Life Events, Social-Support Networks, and Gerontological Health

The following hypotheses are postulated:

1. Poor health status (X_2) will have a direct positive effect on physician visits (X_1), controlling for the effect of prior physician visits (X_3).
2. Physician visits (X_3) will have a direct negative effect on poor health status (X_2), holding prior health status, life events, and social support networks constant.
3. Life events (X_5) experienced in 1969–1971 will adversely affect health status (X_2), controlling for the effect of prior health status, physician visit, and social support networks.
4. Social support networks (X_6) will have a direct negative effect on life events (X_5), poor health (X_2), and physician visits (X_3), and it will also have an indirect effect via poor health on physician visits in 1974 (X_1).

Of primary interest is the relative impact of life events and social-support networks on gerontological health. The present analysis of panel data is restricted to those who had complete information on all of the four waves of the Retirement History Study (N = 4,748). The results of path analysis are presented in the following sections.

Causal Effect of Health Status on Use

Multiple-regression techniques were used to examine the causal effect of prior health status on use of physician services when other factors including life events, social-support networks, SES and prior utilization were simultaneously controlled. The inclusion of prior utilization as a control variable means that panel analysis is performed.

Table 7–1 displays the results of panel regression analyses of physician visits in 1972 and 1974. In the first panel analysis, the prior use of physician visits (1970) is the only significant factor accounting for the variation in the number of physician visits in 1972. Poor health in 1971 had no direct impact on use of physician visits when other factors were considered. (Poor health is operationally defined as a person who had a functional disability or limitation due to illness or injury and also assessed his health as worse than others of his own age.) In the second panel analysis, both poor health measured in 1973 and life events experienced in 1969–1971 had a direct positive effect on use of physician services in 1974, when the effects of the prior use behavior (1972), SES, and social support networks were controlled. The fact that health status in an earlier period (1971) had no impact on the utilization variable but that health in a later period (1973) had a strong direct effect may be explained by two factors. First, the study population was initially restricted to people who were working and had no chronic condition or disability in 1969; therefore, the variation in use of physician services could not be attributed to health-status differences. Second, 7.5 percent of the study population experienced ill health in 1971, and 13.5 percent did in 1973. The increase of physical illness of the panel may explain why the health variable in 1973 exerts a strong positive effect on the use of physician services.

Causal Effect of Stressful Life Events on Physician Use and Health Status

Previous research has indicated that increased stressful life events (SLE) are associated with health-seeking behavior [36, 37]. We examined this relationship by employing a panel regression analysis of physician utilization in 1974 (see table 7-1). The decomposition of effects of stressful life events on poor health and use variables is presented in table 7-2. Controlling for the effect of prior health, physician-use behavior, and other social factors, we found that life events experienced during the period of 1969-1971 exerted a strong positive effect on physician utilization in 1974: the more life-stress events experienced, the greater the number of physician visits. In addition, we found that stressful life events not only directly affected physician utili-

Table 7-1
Panel Regression-Coefficients of the Effects of Health Status and Other Factors on Physician Visits in 1972 and 1974

	Visits in 1972[a]			Visits in 1974[b]		
Predictors	B	Beta	R^2-change	B	Beta	R^2-change
Prior use	.300*	.292	.084	.178*	.173	.035
Poor health	−.059	−.002	.000	2.379*	.088	.008
Live events	−.009	−.029	.001	.010*	.036	.001
Social-support networks	.005	.002	.000	−.010	−.003	.000
SES	−.002	−.024	.001	.009	.010	.000
Intercept	4.255			3.206		
Total variance explained by the model	.086			.044		
Total sample (N)	(4,745)			(4,745)		
Mean	4.170			4.925		
Standard deviation	8.991			9.245		

[a]The use variable is regressed on prior use (1970), X_4, X_5, X_6, and SES.
[b]The use variable is regressed on X_2, X_3, X_5, X_6, and SES.
*Significant at .05 or lower level.

Table 7-2

Decomposition of Effects of Stressful Life Events (SLE) on Poor Health (PH) in 1973 and on the use of Physician Services in 1974

| Effect | Magnitude | | | |
	Total Association[a]	Direct Effect[b]	Indirect Causal Effect[c]	Noncausal Association[d]
Total effect of SLE on PH	.079			
Direct effect		.082		
Indirect effect			none	
Noncausal association				− .003
Total effect of SLE on use	.040			
Direct effect		.036		
Indirect effect via PH			.007	
Noncausal association				− .001

[a]Total effect = direct effect + direct causal effect + indirect causal effect + noncausal association.

[b]Direct effect is the path coefficient.

[c]Indirect causal effect is the total effect of SLE, via poor health variable, on use of physician services.

[d]This refers to the association of SLE with other sociodemographic or precondition factors such as age, race, sex, and so forth.

zation but also indirectly affected the use of physician services via the poor-health variable. We found that SLE's direct effect (beta = .036) on the use variable is greater than its indirect effect (.007).

Examining the relationship between stressful life events and health status, we found poor health was positively associated with the index of life events (r = .026). Data in table 7-3 show that life events experienced in 1969-1971 had a direct positive effect (beta = .082) on poor health in 1973 when prior health and other factors were controlled. This result indicates that the more stressful life events experienced in later life, the more likely the elderly to report poor physical health.

Effects of Social-Support Networks on Stressful Life Events, Poor Health, and Physician Use

Data in table 7-4 show the effects of social-support networks on SLE, health status, and physician utilization. We found that the index of social-support networks in 1971 had no significant impact on the use of physician services when other factors were controlled. This finding does not necessarily imply that social networks have no relevance in the study of the causal influence of social support on gerontological health. Instead, we should carefully examine the role of social networks as an intervening or mediating

Table 7–3
Panel Regression-Coefficients of the Effects of Use of Physical Services, Life Events, and Other Factors on Health Status in 1973

	Probability of Having Poor Health		
Predictors	B	Beta	R^2-change
Prior health (X_4)	.473*	.363	.136
Physician visits (X_3)	.006*	.147	.028
Life events (X_5)	.001*	.082	.001
Social-support networks (X_6) SES	−.002*	−.060	.004
Intercept	.160		
Total variance explained by the model	.169		
Total sample (N)	(4,745)		
Mean	.136		
Standard deviation	.342		

*Significant at .05 or lower level.

Table 7–4
Decomposition of Effects of Social-Support Networks (SS) on Stressful Life Events (SLE) and the Use of Physician Services

	Magnitude			
Effect	Total Association[a] (r)	Direct Effect[b] (p)	Indirect Causal Effect[c]	Noncausal Association[d]
Total effect of SS on use	−.003			
Direct effect		−.005		
Indirect effect				
via PH			.0026	
via SLE			−.0015	
via SLE and PH			−.0004	
Noncausal association				.0013
Total effect of SS on SLE	−.087			
Direct effect		−.050	none	
Noncausal association				−.037
Total effect of SS on PH	.026			
Direct effect		.030		
Indirect effect				
via SLE			−.004	
Noncausal association				none

[a]Total effect = direct effect + indirect causal effect + noncausal effect.

[b]Direct causal effect is the path coefficient.

[c]Indirect causal effect is the total effect of SS via other paths (variables) on an endogenous variable.

[d]This refers to the association of SS with other sociodemographic variables (for example, age, sex, race, SES, and so forth).

factor between stress and ill health. A path diagram based upon panel regression analyses is presented for this purpose (figure 7–2).

The social-support networks (SS) variable had a direct negative effect on SLE. The stronger the social networks, the fewer the stressful life events one will experience in later life. Since SLE is directly related to poor health and physician use, it is clear that the social-support networks may serve as an important factor to mitigate the adverse effect of stressful life events on gerontological health. Inspection of data in figure 7–2 reveals that the magnitude of social-support networks varies by race, sex, and SES. (Males, whites, and people with a low SES are more likely to have a strong network than are females, nonwhites, and those with a high SES.)

There is a positive association between social-support networks and poor health. Careful analysis of data reveals that people who had a strong social network also had poor health initially in the period of 1971. It is likely that a person's ill health may demand more social support from both informal and formal sources; therefore, we find that social-support networks are directly associated with poor health in later periods of their lives.

Discussion

This chapter has presented evidence from panel regression analysis of factors affecting gerontological health. The data seem to lend strong support to our central thesis that cumulative stressful life events have an etiological link with ill health and illness behavior (number of physician visits). When prior health and other factors were taken into account in the panel analysis, a direct, positive relationship was still found between life events and a decline in gerontological health.

The role of social-support networks as a buffering factor between life stress and gerontological health deserves further discussion. We found social-support networks had a negligible effect on physician use. They, however, had a direct, negative influence on stressful life events. We might find a reduction in the deleterious effect of life-change events on health in the context of a social environment conducive to stress reduction or one that provides coping resources for the frail and elderly.

Several measurement problems are likely to be encountered in using a secondary source of data. One is the problem of identifying all of the pertinent life-change events experienced by older adults in retirement. This problem is compounded by the difficulty in employing a universally applicable procedure for weighing the stressful life events. Although the present study has adopted the scaling procedure developed by Holmes and Rahe [5] for eight life events, we do not intend to suggest that their weighting scheme will be perfectly fitted for the study of the elderly population. Further work

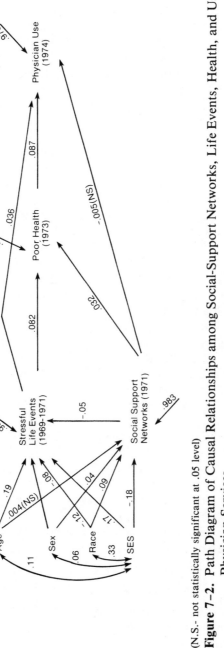

(N.S.- not statistically significant at .05 level)

Figure 7–2. Path Diagram of Causal Relationships among Social-Support Networks, Life Events, Health, and Use of Physician Services.

needs to be done to develop a more valid and reliable life-event schedule to be used specifically for gerontological research.

Another problem is related to the measurement of health, especially for a noninstitutionalized elderly group. Recent research on the validity of viewing health as a complete state of physical, mental, and social well-being has indicated the importance of including personal perceptions (subjective measures) and actual functional capacities (objective measures) in the construction of a health index [38, 39, 40]. Future research on gerontological health should consider the issues of stability and the validity of developing a composite index of health to portray the total configuration.

References

1. Dohrenwend, B.S., "Life Events as Stressors: A Methodological Inquiry," *Journal of Health and Social Behavior* 14 (1973):167–175.

2. Myers, J.K.; J.J. Lindenthal; and M. Pepper, "Life Events and Mental Status: A Longitudinal Study," *Journal of Health and Social Behavior* 13 (1972):398–450.

3. Pesznecker, B.L., and J. McNeil, "Relationship Among Health Habits, Social Assets, Psychological Well-Being, Life Change and Alterations in Health Status," *Nursing Research* 24 (1975):442–447.

4. Rahe, R.H., et al., "Social Stress and Illness Onset," *Journal of Psychosomatic Research* 8 (1964):35–44.

5. Holmes, T.H., and R.H. Rahe, "The Social Readjustment Rating Scale," *Journal of Psychosomatic Research* 11 (1967):213–218.

6. Wyler, A.R.; J. Masuda; and T.H. Holmes, "Magnitude of Life Events and Seriousness of Illness," *Psychosomatic Medicine* 33 (1971): 115–120.

7. Rabkin, J., and E.L. Struening, "Life Events, Stress, and Illness," *Science* 194 (1976):1010–1020.

8. Riley, M.W., and A. Foner, *Aging and Society, Vol. 1: An Inventory of Research Findings* (New York: Russell Sage Foundation, 1968).

9. Atchley, R., *The Social Forces in Later Life* (Belmont, Calif.: Wadsworth Publishing Co., 1972).

10. Katz, S., and A. Akpom, "A Measure of Primary Sociobiological Functions," *International Journal of Health Services* 6 (1976):493–508.

11. Kutner, B., et al., *Five Hundred Over Sixty* (New York: Russell Sage Foundation, 1956).

12. Pihlblad, C., and D. Adams, "Widowhood, Social Participation and Life Satisfaction," *Aging and Human Development* 3 (1972):323–330.

13. Clark, M., and B. Anderson, *Culture and Aging* (Springfield, Ill.: C.C. Thomas, 1967).

14. Streib, G., and C. Schneider, *Retirement in American Society* (Ithaca, New York: Cornell University Press, 1971).

15. Thompson, T.B., "Work Versus Leisure Roles: An Investigation of Morale Among Employed and Retired Men," *Journal of Gerontology* 28 (1973):339–344.

16. Portnoi, V.A., "The Natural History of Retirement," *Journal of the American Medical Association* 245 (1981):1752–1754.

17. Jacobson, D., "Rejection of the Retired Role: A Study of Female Industrial Workers and Their Future," *Human Relations* 20 (1974):477–492.

18. Chatfield, W.F., "Economic and Sociological Factors Influencing Life Satisfaction of the Aged," *Journal of Gerontology* 32 (1977):593–599.

19. Cassel, J., "Physical Illness in Response to Stress," in S. Levine and N. Scotch, eds., *Social Stress* (New York: Aldine Publishing Co., 1970), pp. 189–209.

20. Holmes, T.H., and M. Masuda, "Life Change Illness Susceptibility," in B.P. Dohrenwend and B.S. Dohrenwend, eds., *Stressful Life Events* (New York: John Wiley and Sons, 1974).

21. Ruch, L.O., and T.H. Holmes, "Scaling of Life Change: Comparison of Direct and Indirect Methods," *Journal of Psychosomatic Research* 15 (1970):221–227.

22. Chiriboga, D.A., "Life Event Weighting Systems: A Comparative Analysis," *Journal of Psychosomatic Research* 21 (1977):415–422.

23. Paykel, E.S., "Life Stress and Psychiatric Disorders: Applications of the Clinical Approach," in B.S. Dohrenwend and B.P. Dohrenwend, eds., *Stressful Life Events: Their Nature and Effects* (New York: John Wiley and Sons, 1974).

24. Markush, R.E., and R.V. Favero, "Epidemiological Assessment of Stressful Life Events, Depressed Mood, and Psychophysiological Symptoms: A Preliminary Report," in B.P. Dohrenwend and B.S. Dohrenwend, eds., *Stressful Life Events: Their Nature and Effects* (New York: John Wiley and Sons, 1974), pp. 171–190.

25. Theorell, T., "Life Events Before and After the Onset of a Premature Myocardial Infarction," in B.P. Dohrenwend and B.S. Dohrenwend, eds., *Stressful Life Events* (New York: John Wiley and Sons, 1974).

26. Rahe, R.H., "The Pathway Between Subjects' Recent Life Changes and Their Near-Future Illness Reports: Representative Results and Methodological Issues," in B.P. Dohrenwend and B.S. Dohrenwend, eds., *Stressful Life Events* (New York: John Wiley and Sons, 1974).

27. Cobb, S., "A Model for Life Events and Their Consequences," in B.P. Dohrenwend and B.S. Dohrenwend, eds., *Stressful Life Events* (New York: John Wiley and Sons, 1974).

28. Lin, N.; R.S. Simione; W.M. Ensel; and Wen Kuo, "Social Sup-

port, Stressful Life Events, and Illness: A Model and an Empirical Test,'' *Journal of Health and Social Behavior* 20 (1979):108–109.

29. Cobb, S., "Social Support as a Moderator of Life Stress," *Psychosomatic Medicine* 38 (1976):300–314.

30. Nuckolls, K.B., et al., "Psychological Assets, Life Crisis and the Prognosis of Pregnancy," *American Journal of Epidemiology* 95 (1972): 431–441.

31. Gore, S., "The Effects of Social Support in Moderating the Health Consequences of Unemployment," *Journal of Health and Social Behavior* 19 (1978):157–165.

32. Lowenthal, M., and C. Haven, "Interaction and Adaptation: Intimacy as a Critical Variable," *American Sociological Review* 33 (1968): 20–30.

33. Miller, P.M.; J.G. Ingham; and S. Davidson, "Life Events, Symptoms, and Social Support," *Journal of Psychosomatic Medicine* 20 (1976): 515–522.

34. DeAraujo, G., et al., "Life Change, Coping Ability, and Chronic Intrinsic Asthma," *Journal of Psychosomatic Research* 17 (1973):359–363.

35. Eaton, W.W., "Life Events, Social Supports, and Psychiatric Symptoms: A Re-analysis of New Haven Data," *Journal of Health and Social Behavior* 19 (1978):230–234.

36. Blazer, D., "Life Events, Mental Health Functioning and the Use of Health Care Services by the Elderly," *American Journal of Public Health* 70, no. 11 (1980):1174–1179.

37. Gove, W.R., "Does Help-Seeking Increase Psychological Distress?" *Journal of Health and Social Behavior* 20 (1978):201–202.

38. Tessler, R.; D. Mechanic; and M. Dimond, "The Effect of Psychological Distress on Physician Utilization: A Prospective Study," *Journal of Health and Social Behavior* 17 no. 4 (1976):353–364.

39. Wan, T.T.H.; B.G. Odell; and D.T. Lewis, *Promoting the Well-Being of the Elderly: A Community Diagnosis.* (New York: Haworth Press, 1982).

40. Chappell, N.L., "Measuring Functional Ability and Chronic Conditions Among the Elderly," *Journal of Health and Social Behavior* 22 (March 1982):90–102.

41. Stewart, A.L.; J.E. Ware; and R.H. Brook, "Advances in the Measurement of Functional Status: Construction of Aggregate Indexes," *Medical Care* 19, no. 5 (1981):473–488.

8

Factors Affecting Use of Health Services

When factors affecting the use of health services are evaluated, utilization is usually measured by whether the individual has seen a physician in a specific period prior to the interview and by the number of physician contacts. The evaluation may also take into account incidence and rate of hospitalization.

The factors affecting use of health services have been found to be multiple and diverse in nature [1, 2, 3, 4]. Suchman [5] describes the individual decision to seek health care as occurring in progressive stages. First, there is an awareness of symptoms, which, in turn, leads the individual to define himself as ill. This self-labeling is followed by a decision to go or not to go for care.

Zola [6] identifies five "triggers" that may activate the decision to seek care. These include interpersonal crisis, interference with valued social activity, sanctioning by others, threat to major activity, and nature and familiarity of symptoms.

As mentioned in chapter 1, the popular Andersen [7] model groups the determinants of use of health services into three categories: predisposing, enabling, and need factors. Predisposing factors include demographic, social structural, and attitudinal factors of health beliefs. Enabling factors include family income, insurance benefits, access to care, and availability of community services. Both perceived need, which is subjectively evaluated by the patient, and professionally evaluated need are included in this model. The purpose of this chapter is to present differentials and trends in use of health services. The effect of predisposing, enabling, and need factors is also examined.

Related Research

Predisposing Factors

While the overall number of ambulatory physician visits per person per year has remained at about five visits since 1970 [8], there are variations in number of visits among age, sex, and racial groups. The number of physician visits per person increases with age. This is generally attributed to the higher prevalence of chronic disease among the elderly population. During 1977 the frequency of doctor visits increased with individual age from an average of 4.1 visits per year for children under seventeen years to 6.5 visits per year for people sixty-five and over [9].

Not only are the elderly higher consumers of ambulatory physician services, they have a higher rate of use of acute-care and long-term care facilities. In an examination of the use of acute-care hospital services on an international basis, discharge rates and mean length of stays increased with age in all of the industrialized countries studied [10]. In 1977, 86 percent of nursing-home residents in the United States were over 65 [9].

Sex of the individual accounts for some variation in the use of health services. In 1975, for all adult age groups, females made visits to the doctors at higher rates than did males [8]. According to Mechanic [11], existing data from health examination surveys suggest that much of the excess chronic illness reported by women compared to men is partially a reflection of how they respond to and define illness and their life situation.

Men are less likely to be hospitalized than women throughout young adulthood and middle age [8]. This holds true even when hospitalization for pregnancy and childbirth is taken into account. After the age of fifty-five, men have a higher rate of hospitalization than do women [8]. This may be related to higher incidence of certain chronic diseases, such as heart disease, among men.

Men and women between the ages of sixty-five and seventy-four have almost equal likelihood of institutionalization in a nursing home, but in more advanced age, women are institutionalized at a higher rate than are men [8]. This may be due to the fact that women are more likely than men to be widowed and living alone in later life, and there is an almost twice as high proportion of the widowed among the institutionalized elderly than in the community [12].

Some racial differences in utilization rates have also been noted. According to 1975 data based on the National Health Interview Survey, in all age groups except forty-five to sixty-four years, whites had a higher rate of physician visits than all others [8].

There are racial differences in use of short-stay hospitals. Between 1972 and 1977 black people went from 5 percent fewer discharges per 1,000 to 9 percent greater discharges [9]. The average length of stay was also longer for blacks.

Blacks have a much lower usage of nursing homes than do whites. This may, in part, be related to the discrepancy in life expectancy between blacks and whites. In 1977, the average life expectancy for whites was 73.8; for all other racial groups it was 68.8 [9].

Battistella [13] studied factors associated with delay in the initiation of physician care among the over forty-five. He found that people with positive attitudes toward their health and the efficacy of medicine delay less than do those with unfavorable attitudes. Likelihood of delay also increased with age. This age-related increase in delay of care may mean that the elderly are more skeptical about preventive medical care, and may consider health problems an unavoidable aspect of the aging process [14].

Enabling Factors

In the past, large differences between poor and nonpoor could be seen in the health-services-utilization rate, with the poor using fewer services. Since 1964, there has been a narrowing of the difference between poor and non-poor use of health services [10]. Much of this narrowing has been attributed to the advent of Medicare and Medicaid in 1965.

The gap between elderly poor and nonpoor was slower in narrowing, especially for the elderly nonwhite poor [10]. This trend may reflect the nature of the Medicaid and Medicare programs: Medicaid was designed to serve the low-income population of all ages, while, on the other hand, the Medicare program was designed to benefit people of all incomes who were sixty-five and over [15].

The importance of insurance as an enabling factor has already been shown with the role of Medicaid and Medicare in reducing the inequity between economic groups in access to health services. In a study by Gon-nella et al. [16], it was found that hospitalized patients not covered by com-mercial insurance or Medicaid had significantly more complications than did those who were covered. This difference was thought to reflect lack of access to quality ambulatory care.

In a study of elderly citizens in Baltimore County, Maryland, Wan and Odell [3] found that insurance coverage was not related to use of ambula-tory physician or hospital services. However, participation in a prepaid health plan appeared to reduce the likelihood of hospitalization. This may reflect the preventive-care emphasis of most prepaid plans.

In order to have access to health services, people must be aware of their availability. In a study of Canadian elderly taking into consideration health status, income, and health-service awareness, Snider [17] found that aware-ness was the most important factor in explaining use of health services among the study population.

Need for Care

The need for care, that is, the presence of an illness or poor-health condi-tion, has been found to be the primary factor influencing the decision to see a doctor [7, 11, 18, 19]. In a study of 2,168 households in five New York and Pennsylvania counties, eighteen variables, including individual and community characteristics, were selected to determine the causal ordering of these variables in predicting use of physician services [19]. The need for care, measured by the proportion of household members who have health disorders and who respond to their illness, was the strongest direct causal variable for predicting physician use. It was also found that the need for care was an intermediate factor through which the enabling and predisposing factors affect the course of health actions.

Andersen [7] developed a behavioral systems model of health-services by families. It is a three-stage model that assumes that, in order for health services to be used, (1) a family must be predisposed to receive medical care; (2) enabling conditions allow the family to attain health services; and (3) the family must perceive a need for the service. The combined-need measures explained more of the variation than did the predisposing or enabling factors.

Data collected through personal interviews of 626 families from a sample of employees in a single assembly-manufacturing plant were analyzed to ascertain the roles of need, access, and price as predictors of illness and preventive ambulatory visits [20]. The employees had a choice between three full-coverage HMO-type health plans and Blue Cross-Blue Shield insurance. The findings clearly showed that acute and chronic conditions and perceived health status were the most powerful predictors of the number of visits.

Using a path-analytic technique, Andersen and Aday [21] analyzed a data set based on a national survey of the noninstitutionalized population of the United States conducted by the Center for Health Administration Studies and the National Opinion Research Center of the University of Chicago. The need-variables, measured by number of symptoms reported and by perceived health, were shown to be the prime determinants of the number of physician visits.

In a study of the use of health services among elders, German et al. [22] found, among a population of inner-city elderly, that the majority (over 80 percent) of those reporting the presence of a chronic disease were receiving care. In a study of Boston elders, Branch [23] found that those with the highest level of frailty had higher rates of frequent physician visits than those classified as not frail (a mean of 13.3, compared to 2.4). For a sample of elderly residing in Baltimore County, Maryland, the Andersen model was applied [24]. Need for care was found to be of primary importance in explaining use of physician services and hospitalization.

Analysis of Data

Differentials in Use of Health Services

Data in table 8–1 show that the average number of physician visits for persons in or near retirement age was lower than would be expected (4.9, com-

Table 8-1
Physician Visits in 1970, 1972, and 1974, by Race and Sex

| Year | Average Number of Physician Visits | | | | | Proportion of Persons Having Seen a Physician | | | | |
	Total	White male	White female	Nonwhite male	Nonwhite female	Total	White male	White female	Nonwhite male	Nonwhite female
1970 (N = 5,385)	4.4	4.2	3.8	4.8	4.8	48.7	47.5	45.7	53.0	52.6
1972 (N = 5,107)	4.3	4.2	3.9	4.7	4.4	52.1	51.7	45.8	56.1	48.8
1974 (N = 4,745)	4.9	4.7	5.4	5.4	6.2	57.5	56.2	57.7	61.7	57.9

pared with 6.5). This may be attributed to the fact that, at the first wave (1969) of LRHS data, only those in good health and working were included. The elimination of those with chronic or disabling conditions may account for the low use of physician services. Overall, very little change in the mean number of physician visits throughout the three periods was observed. The only exception is 1974, where a slight increase in the mean is noted.

In all years except 1972, retirees had slightly more physician visits than did workers. The largest difference between retirees and workers in mean physician visits occurred in 1970 (table 8-2). For those who retired during the period of 1969-1971, the advent of an illness episode may have been the precipitating factor in the retirement decision. It is poor health, rather than retirement, that directly affects use of physician services. This is confirmed from a multivariate analysis. We found that retirement had no effect on use, controlling for health, prior use, and other social demographic factors. (Detailed results from panel regression-analyses can be obtained from the author.)

Nonwhites consistently had more physician visits than had whites for all three study years, with the highest level of visits for both groups in 1974 (table 8-1). No discernable pattern of use is evident with nonwhite males and females. In 1972 nonwhite males had more visits than nonwhite females had, but in 1974 the reverse pattern was found. In 1970 and 1972 white females had fewer physician visits than had white males, but by 1974, white females had more visits than white males had. In 1974, both white and nonwhite females had more physician visits.

Nonwhite males were more likely to have seen a physician for all three years than was any other group (table 8-1). No other trends of physician visitation among race/sex groups can be noted. In 1970 and 1974, the precentage of retirees who were visited by a physician was greater than that of workers, but in 1972 the percentage was the same for both (table 8-2).

These unexpected patterns of use of physician services (nonwhites using more physician services and females with fewer visits in some years) can probably by attributed to the study sample. The females included in the sample were nonmarried, working women and only about 11 percent of the study population was nonwhite. Therefore, it would be difficult to make any generalizations to other populations of these specific findings.

In each study year there is a gradual increase in the proportion seeing a physician (forty-nine percent in 1970, compared to fifty-eight percent in 1974). Also, by race/sex and retirement status, the highest number of physician visits were in 1974, when the study population was the oldest for all groups. Clearly, the aging process itself appears to be a factor affecting use of health services. There is a similar trend of increased use of hospital services with each subsequent study period (table 8-3). Time one (1970) had an unusually low percentage of hospitalized people (2.9 percent). Again, this

Table 8-2
Use of Physician Services in 1970, 1972, and 1974, by Retirement Status in 1971

Retired	Total	Retired	Working
		Retirement Status in 1971	
		Average Number of Physician Visits	
1970 (N = 5,385)	4.35	5.67	39.3
1972 (N = 5,107)	4.32	4.03	4.21
1974 (N = 4.745)	4.92	5.29	4.82
		Percentage Having a Physician Visit	
1970	49	52	47
1972	52	52	52
1974	58	61	54

Table 8-3
Proportion of Persons Hospitalized in 1970, 1972, and 1974, by Race and Sex

Year	Total	White male	White female	Nonwhite male	Nonwhite female
1970	2.9	3.1	2.5	2.2	2.2
1972	12.3	13.1	7.5	11.8	7.8
1974	13.8	14.2	11.7	13.6	9.9

was probably because the initial study population was in good health, thus lowering the risk of hospitalization for the total sample. In every period, retirees were more likely to be hospitalized than were workers. As would be expected, males in the age group were hospitalized more often than females and white males were slightly more at risk than nonwhite males.

There is an obvious trend of increased use of both types of health services (physician and hospital) as the study population ages. Being male and retired was also associated with use of hospital services for all three study years (table 8-4).

Table 8-4
Proportions of Persons Hospitalized in 1970, 1972, and 1974, by Retirement Status in 1971

	Retirement Status in 1971		
Year	*Total*	*Retired*	*Working*
1970	2.9	4.03	2.51
1972	12.3	13.1	10.4
1974	13.8	14.2	12.4

Relative Importance of Factors Affecting
Health-Services Utilization

The effect of predisposing, enabling, and need factors on use of health services is examined by a panel regression analysis, using the number of physician visits and the probability of hospitalization in 1972 and 1974 as dependent variables (tables 8-5 and 8-6). Predisposing factors include prior use of physician and hospital services, age, SES, sex, race, and a measure of stressful life events. The enabling factor is a measure of social-support networks. The need for care includes decline in self-assessed health and life satisfaction and an increase in the level of disability.

Looking first at the use of physician services in 1972 and 1974 (table 8-5), prior use of physician services, a predisposing variable, is the most significant predictor of use in both years. This finding is expected since previous visit to a physician would indicate a similar pattern of use in later periods. Furthermore, prior use of physician services could indicate the presence of a health condition needing continued care.

Sex, another predisposing factor, was significantly associated with the number of physician visits in 1974, but not in 1972. Women have more visits than do men. This is the expected pattern of use between males and females. Referring to table 8-1, which shows the breakdown of mean number of visits by race/sex, one can see that both white and nonwhite females have a higher number of mean visits than do their male counterparts in 1974.

In 1974, the decline in health in terms of worsening perceived health and increasing disability was significantly associated with an increase in physician visits. The increased significance of these variables as predictors of the use of physician services in the later study period would be expected. At the outset, the total sample was in good health, but, as the cohort aged, one would expect to see an increase in the incidence of health problems, necessitating physician services.

Table 8-5
Panel Regression-Coefficients of the Effects of Predisposing, Enabling, and Need Factors on Number of Physician Visits in 1972 and 1974

| | Number of Physician Visits | | | |
| | 1972 | | 1974 | |
Predictors	B	Beta	B	Beta
Predisposing Factors				
Prior use[a]	0.295*	0.29	0.172*	0.17
Age	0.085	0.02	0.060	0.01
Sex (male = 1; female = 0)	− 0.406	− 0.02	− 0.800*	− 0.04
Race (white = 1; nonwhite = 0)	0.331	0.01	− 0.930	− 0.03
SES	− 0.014	− 0.02	0.017	0.02
Stressful life events[b]	− 0.008	− 0.03	0.006	3.41
Enabling Factor				
Social support	− 0.012	− 0.00	0.008	0.00
Need for Care				
Decline in self-assessed health[c]	− 0.900*	0.03	1.417*	0.05
Decline in life satisfaction[c]	− 0.144	− 0.00	0.093	0.00
Increase in disability[c]	0.410	1.01	1.712*	0.08
R^2	.086		0.052	
Mean	4.3		4.9	
Standard deviation	8.97		9.22	
Total (N)	(5107)		(4622)	

[a]Prior use in 1972 was measured by number of physician visits in 1970, and in 1974 by number of physician visits in 1972.

[b]Stressful life events as a measure for 1972 is a weighted aggregation of events occurring between 1969 and 1971, and for 1974, events occurring between 1969 and 1973.

[c]For 1972, the decline in health and life satisfaction and increase in disability is measured as it occurs between 1969 and 1971; for 1974 the above is measured as it occurs between 1969 and 1973.

*Significant at .05 or lower level

Of primary importance in explaining hospitalization in 1972 and 1974 (table 8–6) is prior hospitalization. A previous hospitalization could indicate the presence of an ongoing health problem and possible future hospital stays. An increase in disability, a direct measure of need in care, was significantly related to hospitalization in both years. Everything else being equal, whites were significantly more likely to be hospitalized than were nonwhites.

Discussion

There is no discernable pattern of use of health services in the panel study. Although retirement occurring in 1969–1971 was positively associated with

Stressful Life Events

Table 8-6
Panel Regression-Coefficients of the Effects of Predisposing, Enabling, and Need Factors on Hospitalization in 1972 and 1974

| | Hospitalized | | | |
| | 1972 | | 1974 | |
Predictors	B	Beta	B	Beta
Predisposing Factors				
Prior use[a]	0.12*	0.07	0.64*	0.06
Age	0.69	0.01	−0.15	−0.01
Sex (male = 1; female = 0)	1.05	0.01	0.49	0.01
Race (white = 1; nonwhite = 0)	5.32*	0.05	1.77	0.01
SES	0.10	0.01	0.87	0.03
Stressful life events[b]	0.17	0.02	0.42	0.01
Enabling Factor				
Social support	0.22	0.02	−0.18	−0.00
Need for Care				
Decline in self-assessed health[c]	0.83	0.01	−0.39	−0.00
Decline in life satisfaction[c]	−0.34	−0.00	−0.25	−0.11
Increase in disability[c]	3.32*	0.04	5.03*	0.07
R^2		.01		.01
Mean		12.30		13.76
Standard deviation				
Total (N)				

[a]Prior use in 1972 was measured by hospitalization in 1970, and in 1974 by hospitalization in 1972.

[b]Stressful life events, as a measure for 1972, is a weighted aggregation of events occurring between 1969 and 1971, and for 1974, events occurring between 1969 and 1973.

[c]For 1972, the decline in health and life satisfaction and increase in disability is measured as it occurs between 1969 and 1971; for 1974 the above is measured as it occurs between 1969 and 1973.

*Significant at .05 or lower level.

use of health services, the differences in health-services use between retirees and workers disappear when health status, prior use, age, and other demographic factors are controlled. This finding suggests that retirement has no significant impact on the use of health services.

After careful inspection of health-services use in 1970, 1972, and 1974, we find a definite trend of increased use of services for each successive period as the cohort ages.

Neither a cross-sectional study nor a retrospective study can clearly demonstrate the causal relationship between predictors and the use of health services the way that a prospective study can. A complete model of determinants of use of health services cannot be examined without having specific information about the awareness of services available in the community, the accessibility to care, and other enabling factors. This information was not available in the LRHS data. Nonetheless, this area should be pursued in the future within a prospective framework.

References

1. Andersen, R., and J.F. Newman, "Societal and Individual Determinants Medical Care Utilization in the United States," *The Milbank Memorial Fund Quarterly* 51 (1973):95-124.

2. Berki, S.E., and B. Kobashigawa, "Socioeconomic and Need Determinants of Ambulatory Care Use: Path Analysis of the 1970 Health Interview Survey Data," *Medical Care* 14 (1976):405-421.

3. Wan, T.T.H., and B.G. Odell, "Factors Affecting the Use of Social and Health Services Among the Elderly," *Aging and Society* 1, no. 1 (1981):95-115.

4. Wan, T.T.H., "Access to Care and Health Services Utilization by the Elderly in Low-Income Communities," *Milbank Memorial Fund Quarterly* 60 (Winter 1982):137-151.

5. Suchman, E.A., "Stages of Illness and Medical Care," *Journal of Health and Human Behavior* 6 (1965):2-16.

6. Zola, I.K., "Culture and Symptoms: An Analysis of Patients Presenting Complaints," *American Sociological Review* 31 (1966):615-630.

7. Anderson, R., *A Behavioral Model of Families Use of Health Service* (Chicago, Ill.: University of Chicago, Center for Health Administration Studies, Research Series 27, 1968).

8. U.S. Department of Health, Education and Welfare, *Health, United States, 1976-1977,* Publication No. (HRA), (1977), pp. 77-1232.

9. U.S. Department of Health, Education and Welfare, *Health, United States, 1979,* Publication No. (PHS), (1979), pp. 80-1232.

10. U.S. Department of Health and Human Services, *Health, United States, 1980,* Publication No. (PHS), (1980), pp. 81-1232.

11. Mechanic, D., "Sex, Illness, Illness Behavior, and the Use of Health Services," *Journal of Human Stress* 2 (1976):29-40.

12. Shanas, E., "The Family as a Social Support System in Old Age," *The Gerontologist* 19 (1979):169-174.

13. Battistella, R.N., "Factors Associated with Delay in the Initiation of Physicians' Care Among Late Adulthood Persons," *American Journal of Public Health* 61 (1971):1348-1361.

14. Riley, M., and A. Foner, *Aging and Society, Vol. 1.* (New York: Russell Sage Foundation, 1968).

15. Aday, L.; R. Andersen; and G.V. Fleming, *Health Care in the U.S.* (Beverly Hills, Calif.: Sage Publications, Inc., 1980).

16. Gonnella, J.S.; D.Z. Louis; and J.C. McCord, "The Staging Concept: An Approach to the Assessment of Outcome of Ambulatory Care," *Medical Care* 14, no. 1 (1976):13–21.

17. Snider, E.L., "Awareness and Use of Health Services by the Elderly," *Medical Care* 18 (1980):1177–1182.

18. Richardson, W.C., "Measuring the Urban Poors Use of Physician Services in Response to Illness Episodes," *Medical Care* 8 (1970):132–142.

19. Wan, T.T.H., and S.J. Soifer, "Determinants of Physician Utilization: A Causal Analysis," *Journal of Health and Social Behavior* 15 (1974): 100–108.

20. Berki, S.E., and M.L. Ashcraft, "On the Analysis of Ambulatory Utilization," *Medical Care* 17 (1979):1163–1180.

21. Andersen, R., and L.A. Aday, "Access to Medical Care in the U.S.: Realized and Potential," *Medical Care* 16 (1978):533–546.

22. German, P.S.; E.A. Skinner; and S. Shapiro, "Ambulatory Care for Chronic Conditions in an Inner City Elderly Population," *American Journal of Public Health* 66 (1976):660–666.

23. Branch, L.G., *Boston Elders: A Survey of Needs 1978.* (Boston, Mass.: Center for Survey Research, A Facility of the University of Massachusetts, the Joint Center for Urban Studies of M.I.T., Harvard University and the Boston Urban Observatory of the University of Massachusetts, 1978).

24. Wan, T.T.H.; D.L. Lewis; and B.G. Odell, *Senior Needs Assessment Project* (University of Maryland Baltimore County, Department of Sociology, as contracted by Baltimore County Department of Aging, 1980).

9 Summary and Conclusions

In the literature on social precursors of ill health evidence has shown that social stress, induced by frequent life changes or role losses, may make an individual susceptible to physical and mental illness. Therefore, we postulated that illness or illness behavior (physician utilization) is positively associated with the magnitude of life events experienced in later life. Based on four waves (1969, 1971, 1973, and 1975) of the Longitudinal Retirement History Study, we identified eight major life events pertaining to changes in work status, marital status, living arrangement, family relationship, and economic status of older adults, and examined their relative influences on health and health-care use. In additiion, we investigated the role of social-support networks as buffering factors between life events and gerontological health. A prospective study design was employed to follow up a panel of working older adults who had no physical incapacities or disabling conditions in the initial study period. Panel regression analysis was performed to determine the causal effects of life events and social-support networks on gerontological health, while the prior health status and other sociodemographic factors were simultaneously controlled.

Major findings and their implications from this investigation can be summarized as follows.

First, the validity of three interrelated dimensions of health (physical disability, life satisfaction, and self-assessed health) was evaluated by a multiple-indicator model in order to derive estimates of stability coefficients across the three waves of panel data. The results indicate that the stability coefficients increase over time; the assessment of general health does not change very much over a four-year period. The health variable, measured by life satisfaction, is less reliable than are self-assessed health and disability. In order to validate the predictive value of the three health indicators, life events, mortality status, and the use of health services were regressed on each of these indicators. We found that health indicators had a direct positive effect on the magnitude of life events, the use of health services, and mortality status: Those in poor health would be more likely to experience stressful major life events, use more health services, and have a higher risk of mortality in later life.

With knowledge about the validity and stability of health indicators, researchers need to further identify measurement errors of health variables. Future studies should include (1) specification of causal directions of various health status indicators; (2) assessment of the amount of variation in objective measures of physical health accounted for by certain subjective measures, such as perceived health, life satisfaction, and other personal evaluation of health status; and (3) development of a universally applicable index of health for studying noninstitutionalized elders.

Second, role loss constitutes a life event that might be expected to have a deleterious effect on gerontological health. This assumption was empirically validated by panel regression analyses. Controlling for the prior health status of the elderly we found that retirement, per se, had no significant effect on health. Of the five role losses studied, widowhood was the most important predictor of poor health. This provides some empirical evidence that widowhood is a stressful life event adversely affecting the sense of well-being of the elderly. Furthermore, our analysis also suggests that the relationship of role loss to health may be ascertained by examining the cumulative experience of multiple role losses in a specified period.

Third, all persons in our study sample appear to have some form of social-support networks, regardless of race, sex, marital status, and living arrangement. With the exception of widowhood, role losses had a negligible effect on the magnitude of social-support networks.

Fourth, based on social-stress theories, life events should be weighted in accordance with their relative importance in affecting the adaptation. We singled out eight major life events including role loss variables, declining economic status, and the change in living arrangements in a specific period (two years).

We constructed an index using the weighting procedure developed by Holmes and Rahe [1]. Path analytic techniques were applied to investigate the causal effects of stressful life events and social-support networks on health and health services utilization of the panel. The results reveal that the magnitude of life events exerted both a direct and an indirect effect, via the health-status variable, on use of physician services. The social-support network variable had a negligible impact on physician utilization, but it had a strong direct-negative effect on the magnitude of stressful life events experienced in 1969–1971. These findings confirm our initial theoretical assumption that the social-support network, as a contextual variable, mitigates the adverse effect of stressful life events on gerontological health. It might be expected that elderly people who have greater social networks also use the available formal support systems (for example, social and health service networks) more effectively and are less likely to have a decline in health.

The findings of this study have theoretical, methodological and pragmatic relevance for gerontological research and practice.

Theoretically, our study has enhanced our understanding of the relationships among life change, social support, illness, and use of health services. Although previous studies using less sophisticated analytical techniques have demonstrated a relationship among these variables, our analysis of longitudinal data suggest that this relationship is more complex than was originally anticipated. Retirement alone appears to have little impact on health or use of health services. However, our evidence indicates a strong synergistic effect of retirement in combination with other life events. Moreover, our data suggest that social support is viewed most appropriately as a contextual factor that mediates the impact of life events on health, since social-support networks did not have a direct effect on health, but had a negative effect on the amount of life changes experienced. Therefore, while the data do not directly show the mediating or buffering effect of social support in reducing stress from life change, our evidence implies that the primary role played by social-support networks is preventive in nature, reducing the amount of change experienced in the first place. This model of social support merits additional inquiry in future research.

From the methodological perspective, this study also has made several contributions to advancing the development of a panel analysis of the causal relationship between life events and gerontological health. First, the use of four waves of panel data has enabled us to demonstrate causal relationships between the study variables. This prospective approach has eliminated difficulties with memory bias and faulty recall that have plagued many of the previous retrospective studies in this area. In addition, use of panel regression and path analysis has allowed us to ascertain the causal relationships between life change and health while controlling for other extraneous factors. For example, through the use of sophisticated analytical techniques, we were able to determine that the event of retirement had no significant impact on ill health when health status at the initial period of this study was controlled. Thus, we were able to demonstrate that prior health status rather than an event such as retirement is the prime determinant of health of retirees.

Finally, our results with the use of an objectively weighted index of life events tend to validate subjective assessments of the impact of these life events in other studies such as Holmes and Rahe. Both our objective assessment and other subjective assessments confirm that the major role loss, widowhood, requires the greatest psychological adjustment.

From a pragmatic point of view, the findings of our study should prove useful to physicians and others who wish to facilitate their patients' or clients' adjustment to stressful life events in old age. Foremost is our recommendation that retirement be considered a process rather than a static event. Viewed as a process, retirement requires continual adjustment. Our study demonstrates the importance of encouraging preventive health behaviors prior to retirement to enhance health in the retirement years.

Physicians and professionals involved in preretirement planning should make efforts to teach the importance of good health maintenance, since prior health status is a strong determinant of health after retirement. The role of the physician as educator rather than as counselor has been suggested by Portnoi [3]. Second, pre-retirees should be alerted to the importance of maintaining informal social-support networks in later life. Men, especially, need to be aware of the importance of social support in aiding adjustment to life change. In our primarily male study-population, widowhood was the major role loss with the greatest impact on social support. This suggests men rely on their spouse to maintain their informal social network. For these men, the loss of spouse also reduced social supports available outside the home.

While this book does not find that retirement has an adverse impact on health, our data indicate that retirement does occur concomitantly with other life events that may combine to produce a negative effect on health. Greater attention should be given to reducing the occurrence or ameliorating the negative effects of decline in economic status or change in living arrangements.

Further research should be directed toward a continued examination of the long-term effects of major role losses on health and use of services. Our study was limited to the first four waves of the LRHS data, allowing us to follow the retirement process for a period of six years. As the complete set of LRHS data becomes available, a study of retirees over the entire ten-year period will help to clarify the consistency of the trends in this report over a longer period. Also, a longer time-span might allow us to make more accurate determinations of any cohort variations in adjustment to retirement.

While our study has revealed that the relationship among social support, life change, and health is more complex than heretofore realized, more research is required to examine the importance of social support at all stages in the life cycle, and to further define the relationship between social support and life changes. Questions that still need to be addressed include:

1. How important in mediating stress are support networks outside the nuclear family, as compared to relationships within the nuclear unit?
2. Does the breadth or the intensity of social-support networks have the greater impact on coping?
3. What tasks of the social-support network (instrumental or emotional) have the most direct effect on coping, health, and use of health services?

Our study has taken a major step toward unraveling the confounding relationships which exist among life change, social support and health variables. Future research must further clarify these complex interrelationships.

References

1. Holmes, T.H., and R. Rahe, "The Social Readjustment Rating Scale," *Journal of Psychosomatic Research* 11 (1967):213–218.

2. Holmes, T.H., and M. Masuda, "Life Change and Illness Susceptibility," in B.S. Dohrenwend and B.P. Dohrenwend, eds., *Stressful Life Events: Their Nature and Effects* (New York: John Wiley and Sons, 1974).

3. Portnoi, V.A., "The Natural History of Retirement," *Journal of the American Medical Association* 245 (1981):1752–1754.

**Annotated Bibliography:
Stressful Life Events,
Social Support,
and Health**

Author(s) (date)	Sample or Study Design	Measure of Life Change Events	Measure of Social Support	Measure of Health	Findings
Atchley, R. (1975)	902 men and women aged 70–79.	Widowhood	—	—	(1) Widowed were more likely (than married people of the same age) to identify themselves as old and to be lonely. (2) Widowers more likely than widows to increase their level of social participation following retirement. (3) Widowers were more likely to have adequate incomes than widows. (4) The effects of widowhood vary with the industry group considered.
Berardo, F. (1970)	Literature review	Widowhood	—	Mortality, suicide, mental disorder	Widowed have higher mortality, mental disorder, and suicide than married.
Burch, J. (1972)	Suicides $N = 75$ Control $SN = 150$ Aged 21–65+ Matched control	Loss of parent or spouse	—	Suicide (depressive illness	It was hypothesized that there is some causal relation between bereavement of a parent or spouse and suicide of the bereaved person. There was a 5x higher rate of bereavement among suicide groups than control groups. Suicide following bereavement seemed more likely when person had shown a previous tendency to psychiatric breakdown and was not closely supported by a family group.

Blazer, D. (1980)	$N = 186$ aged 65+	16 of the 44 life events of the Holmes and Rahe Schedule of Recent Events were included in a questionnaire. They are death of spouse, personal injury or illness, fired at work, death of a close family member, marital separation, death of a close friend, change in health of a family member, divorce, change in number of arguments with spouse, change in where you live, change in financial state, sex difficulties, retirement, spouse begins or stops work, change in living condition, marriage or remarriage.	—	Mental-health function. The questionnaire about mental health includes items to assess organic brain deficit, personality, life satisfaction, previous use of inpatient and outpatient psychiatric services, and subjective evaluation of mental health status.	(1) 18 subjects (about 10 %) in this study had life change units (LCU's) 150. (2) A crude estimate of the relative risk for mental health impairment given life change events 150 was 2.14. (3) increased life events were associated with health seeking behavior, but the association between increased life events and both mental health functioning and health seeking behavior were small, suggesting that life events may not be important risk factors for elderly living in the community.
Casscels, W., et al. (1980)	$N = 1136$ Aged 30–75 Married white men. 568 men who died from CHD -568 controlled subjects	Retirement	—	Died from coronary heart disease (CHF) within 24 hours. of the onset of symptoms.	After adjustment for age and history of hospitalization for myocardial infarction, the relative risk was reduced to indicate that those who had retired had an 80% greater risk of death from CHF than those who had not. These data suggested that retirement and subsequent coronary mortality may be linked.

Author(s) (date)	Sample or Study Design	Measure of Life Change Events	Measure of Social Support	Measure of Health	Findings
Cobb, S. (1976)	Literature review	—	—	Several measures	Thesis: social support facilitates coping with crisis and adaptation to change. Among studies reviewed supporting this thesis are Nuckolls et al. (1972), which deals with complications in pregnancy, Jessner (1952), which concerns posthospitalization psychological reactions among children; DeAraujo and Van Arsdal (1973), which demonstrates value of social support in reducing need for steroid therapy; Parkes (1972), which reports that support correlates with good psychological adjustment following widowhood.
Cohen, S.I., J. Hajioff (1972)	$N = 52$ $M = 14$ $F = 38$ Aged 35–86 with diagnosed acute closed-angle glaucoma; 52 matched controls from other hospitalized patients. Retrospecive study	History of LCE's in preceding 3 months	—	Incidence of acute closed-angle glaucoma	(1) It was hypothesized that the onset of acute closed-angle glaucoma is related to stress or change in the life situation. (2) Findings of study tend to support the clinical impression that emotional stress plays a part in the etiology of acute closed-angle glaucoma, though not as great a part as earlier literature would suggest.

Crisp, A.H., R.G. Priest (1972)	$N = 777$ $M = 64$ $F = 65$ Aged 40–65 Selected from group practice London Nonrandom systemic selection	Loss of close relative	—	Middlesex Hospital questionnaire—A standard brief self-rating inventory to cover clinical range of neurotic illness	(1) It was hypothesized that there is a relationship between psychoneurotic mobidity to bereavement. (2) Weak results, no clear association.
Croog, S.H. (1972)	$N = 345$ Males aged 30–59 experiencing first myocardial infarction	—	Help received from family and nonkin	Experience of heart attack and recovery	Members of the kin group as well as friends and neighbors ranked similarly in degree of assistance, with kin ranking slightly higher. Very little use of institutional or professional helping service was used side from contact with physician.
Dean, A., et al. (1980)	1091 respondents multi-stage random sample. Ages 17–25 yrs. 50+ years	(1) Checklist of 119 items including those of Holmes and Rahe and Myers et al. (2) respondents evaluated happenings in previous 6 months.	(1) 26-item scale to tap instrumental and emotional support	Cornell Medical Index	(1) Study relates type of support to depression. (2) Findings indicate lack of certain types of support among varying age groups as associated with the occurrence of depression (3) In the old age group (65+) having too many responsibilities, not being married, having illness problems and low income were related to depression.

Author(s) (date)	Sample or Study Design	Measure of Life Change Events	Measure of Social Support	Measure of Health	Findings
DeAraujo, G., et al. (1973)	N = 36 -Chronic intrinsic-asthmatic patients. Panel study	SRE	—	Severity of Chronic Asthma	(1) Hypothesized relationship patients with low psychological assets (measured by Berle Score) and high environmental changes would tend to pursue a more severe course and need higher doses of medication to control diseases. (2) There was no apparent relationship between the SRE score and dosage of medication but when psychosocial assets were included in the evaluation it was found patients with low psychosocial assets and high life change required significantly more medication than those with low assets and low life change. It was clinically observed that patients with low coping ability and high life change were continuously incapacitated.
Eaton, W.W. (1978)	N = 720 Same as Myer's 1972 New Haven Sample Longitudinal Panel data	List developed by Meyers et al. based on Antonovsky and Katz (1967), Holmes and Rahe and additional items	—	Mental Health Index based on Macmillan (1975) and Gurin et al. (1960	(1) It was hypothesized that the availability of social supports lessen the impact of life events on mental disorders. (2) Life events are more stressful for those not accustomed to

them—social supports such as marriage or living with others help absorb the burden of stress and thus help prevent mental disorder.

Study	Sample/Method	Loss/Stress measure	Social support measure	Outcome measure	Findings
Elwell-Maltbie F., Crannell, A.D. (1981)		Measure death of spouse, death of close family member, personal injury or illness, retirement—loss of personal and social resources.	(1) Socializing in informal setting (neighbors and friends), (2) family participation—frequency of socializing (3) formal participation and number of group memberships.	General health status	(1) Effects of role loss more significant for men than women. (2) Men—level of education and roll loss had an effect on health findings. (3) Women—age and educational level have an affect on health. (4) Widowhood's effect on health is indirect, mediated by income status.
Eckenrode, J., Gore, S. (forthcoming)	Random sample of 356 women on registration list of neighborhood health center Prospective study (1 year)	(1) Interviews, T_1 and T_2 (one yr. later). (2) Diaries of health and stress. (3) Report events happening to respondents and family and friends.	Measured two ways: (1) Potential supporters (person who could be called on for help), (2) actual supporters (those who gave help)	(1) Medical Record (2) Provider assessment of psychosocial stress.	Data collection in progress. *Preliminary hypotheses* (1) Study proposes to demonstrate that from a pool of potential supporters, a group of possible supporters is drawn after constraints on potential supporters are taken into account. (2) Study of the context in which support is given (that is, the stresses on potential supporters) is necessary to understand the buffering effects of support on stress.

Author(s) (date)	Sample or Study Design	Measure of Life Change Events	Measure of Social Support	Measure of Health	Findings
Fenwick, R. and Barresi, C.M. (1981)	Longitudinal and cross-sectional analysis of 7696 respondents 65 +; HEW 1973-74 Survey of the low-income aged and disabled.	Change in marital status (1) Married to not married (2) Not married to married	—	(1) Self-perceived health status. (2) Number of days ill in bed at home. (3) Number of days in hospital, nursing home, and other medical institution.	(1) There were clear differences between cross-sectional and longitudinal models in analyzing the effects of marital-status changes on changes in health status; (2) Marital status added significant variance to the *longitudinal study* for perceived health and days in bed, but only to the *cross sectional* equation for perceived health. Those widowed between T1 and T2 had lower perceived health at T2 but fewer days in bed than those in other marital groups; (3) Those who were widowed before T1 had higher rates of institutionalization at T2 showing the possible long term effects of widowhood; (4) Those who never married had better perceived health and spent fewer days ill in bed than married respondents.
Foner, A. and Schwab, R. (1980)	LRHS Data "Does Health Limit Work?" working 169 retired 173 62-67 years.	Retirement	—	Retirement and health	(1) One half sample said health had probably interfered with ability to work. 30% said health kept them from working at all; (2) Some people may try to justify retirement by saying they have poor health; (3) married do better

Author (year)	Sample				Findings
					in retirement—widowed and divorced lack social support.
Fillenbaum, G.G. (1979)	$N = 320$ 120 Community Residents 65 + age. 98 clients at clinic, age 50 +, 192 institutional residents	—	—	—	As person ages inter-dependency among different areas of personal functioning increase.
Finlayson, A (1976)	$N = 76$ females whose husbands survived 12 months after heart attack.	Availability of lay helpers and consultants including family and friends.	—	Recovery of husband from heart attack.	Wives whose husbands had favorable outcomes (husbands at work and wives defining illness as over) tended to be those who acknowledge support from a wider range of sources (friends and family). Conversely, wives whose husbands had less favorable outcomes tended to be those who acknowledged support from a narrower range of sources.
Fuller, S.S., Larson, S.B. (1980)	$N = 50$ Age 51-89	Frequency and magnitude of life events experienced during the preceding 12 months were measured by the Geriatric Schedule of Recent Experience	(1) Measurement was retrospective; (2) Emotional support was selected as one form of social support; (3) A ten-item scale was developed for the measurement of emotional support.	The Guttman Health Scale for the Aged was used for assessment of functional health.	(1) Life events are negatively correlated with functional health and with the agitation dimension of morale. (2) The regression of agitation in life events is conditional on the level of emotional support. But, there is no evidence that emotional support moderates the effects of life events on the index of health. (3) Emotional support is not related significantly to physical health. But, it is related positively to the loneliness dissatisfaction dimension of morale and to the combined-morale index.

Author(s) (date)	Sample or Study Design	Measure of Life Change Events	Measure of Social Support	Measure of Health	Findings
Gelein, J.L. (1980)	Literature review	—	Enduring pattern of continuous or intermittent ties that play a part in maintaining psychological and physical integrity.		(1) Cites Mitchell's (1969) theory of relationship between social support and health: (a) the greater the structural availability of social support, the greater the health protectiveness; (b) greater the support functions, the more health protective the social network; (2) Several animal studies, Conger, 1958; Henry et al., 1967; and human studies, McMiller and Ingham, 1976; Holmes, 1954; support this conclusion; (3) Implications of the review include that health care practitioners should be educated to incorporate concepts of social support into their practice; aging women should develop life styles that incorporate multiple sources of support; stressful situations that include older women should be classified along with possible source of social support.
George, L.K. Maddox, G.L. (1977)	Longitudinal Study—58 male subjects	Retirement	—	—	Psychological adaptation to retirement is conditioned by social resources. Being married and having socioeconomic status facilitates adaptation.

Reference	Sample	Instrument	Variables	Findings
Goldberg, E.L., Comstock, G.W. (1980)	2780 subjects range from 18 years to over 65.	List of forty-one life events based on the work of Holmes and Rahe.	—	(1) 85 percent of events were reported more frequently by people under 45. (2) Men were more likely to report five or more events than women. (3) Separated and divorced persons rank highest in the frequency of life events while never married and married rank lowest. (4) Education was positively related to the number of life events experienced.
Guttman, D. (1978)	$N = 410$; stratified sample average age 71-87 years.	Total 34 life-change events	—	(1) Higher number of events more action taken; (2) education, income and satisfaction with decisions significant in perceiving life events as positive or negative.
Holtzman, M., et al., (1980)	$N = 80$ 45 retirees 35 non-retirees	Early retirement	1–Housing 2–Retired friends 3–Education 4–Income and financial status 5–Job satisfaction 6–Family involvement	Selfreported 1–Health status 2–Health worries 3–Number of recent physician visits 4–Recent history of hospitalization 5–Presence of specific health problems 6–Reduction of daily activities

(1) Early retirees tended to be older, have less formal education, have their own homes free, have less retired friends, have greater health problems, have higher levels of anomia and be more externally oriented, have less job satisfaction and, have lower income. (2) No significant differences between retirees and nonretirees in (1) variables pertaining to family involvement, (2) variables related to financial status, (3) the sources of friends, (4) leisure activities.

Author(s) (date)	Sample or Study Design	Measure of Life Change Events	Measure of Social Support	Measure of Health	Findings
Horwitz, A (1978)	N = 120 white middle class, outpatients and short-term in-patients at a mental health center		Marital Status, availability of kin, including children, parents, and siblings; availability of friends and peers	Mental health	Those with gratifying relationships within the nuclear family do not place high reliance on kin and friends for assistance. Where poor nuclear family relations occur, help sought for mental health problems most often from friends followed closely by parents and siblings. All members of social network provide advice. Services, however, are usually only provided by kin and provision of services is not interchangeable between kin and friends when kin is not available. Friends are more likely than kin to suggest that persons seek professional help.
Hyman, D.K., Gianturco, D.T. (1973)	Longitudinal N = 260 (over 60 years)	Widowhood	—	Health status	(1) Widows experience time related health deterioration only.
Justice, B., et al. (1980)	187 students in professional curriculum of School of Public Health	Recent life changes questionnaire (RLCQ) (Measured events experienced during specific recall periods of 1 year and adjustment associated with events).	20-item scale measuring perceived friendliness of school atmosphere, helpfulness of fellow students, living arrangement, etc.	General well-being	(1) Study failed to find evidence supporting buffering effect of social support.

Kaplan, B.H., Cassel, J.C., Gore, S. (1977)

Literature review and discussion

—

—

—

(1) In both human and animal studies the presence of another animal of same species may protect individuals from stressful stimuli. (2) Description of accessibility criteria is as follows: 1. Anchorage; 2. Reachability—extent person can use of contact people important to him; 3. Range—Number of direct contacts (few or many); 4. Content (meaning given relationship). Directness-reciprocity, Intensity, Frequency.

Kimmel, D.C., Price, K.S., Walker, J.W. (1978)

Recent retirees (within 5 years) U.S. and Canadian corporations. Average age 65.7, 85 percent married

Retirement

—

—

(1) Voluntary retirees: higher income, occupation and health, more family support for decision to retire. (2) Voluntary retirees more likely positive attitude toward retirement. (3) Health status and preretirement feelings strongest predictors of retirement attitudes. (4) Voluntary retirees adjusted better to retirement (average time adjustment 7.1 months), involuntary length of adjustment (12.5 months). (5) Postretirement health status related to attitudes about retired life and satisfaction with retirement.

Author(s) (date)	Sample or Study Design	Measure of Life Change Events	Measure of Social Support	Measure of Health	Findings
Langlie, J. (1977)	N = 383 urban adults	—	Measurement of interaction with kin and nonkin	Preventive Health Behavior—Direct PHB-driving habits, etc. indirect PHB-dental and medical checkups immunization, etc.	Appropriate indirect PHB was associated with control variables, frequent interaction with nonkin; appropriate direct PHB was not significantly associated with interaction on kin or non-kin level.
Lin, N., et al. (1980)	N = 550 Chinese-Americans	Modified version of Holmes and Rahe SRRS	Scale of nine items tapping interaction with friends, neighbors, and the subcultural community and social adjustment.	24-item psychiatric symptom scale (symptoms in the last 6 months before survey).	(1) Presence of stressors is positively related to the incidence of psychiatric symptoms. (2) Social support is negatively related to the presence of psychicatric symptoms than stressful life events.
Linn, M.W., et al. (1980)	N = 188 aged 65+	12 events were assessed. (1) Change of residence, (2) Death of family member or close friend. (3) Serious personal illness. (4) Having a family member or close friend who had experience a serious illness. (5) Change in marital status. (6) Financial problems. (7) Legal problems. (8) Change with		Symptoms of depression were measured by the Depression Factor Score from the Hopkins Symptom Checklist. Scores were divided into two groups, depressed and nondepressed. Will-to-live scale was also used. In addition, subjects were asked whether they used tranquilizers or not.	(1) 25 percent of the 188 subjects were considered depressed. (2) Symptoms of depression were slightly higher in females as opposed to males, and higher in whites as compared with blacks. (3) The most frequently reported events were death of a friend or relative, personal serious illness, illness of a relative or friend, and consequential arguments with family or close friends. (4) The elderly with greater depressive symptomatology had been involved

	in more arguments with friends or family, experienced more deaths of relatives and friends, and among the white elderly, reported more accidents among relatives and friends. (5) The elderly with greater depressive symptomatology were more likely to have experienced greater stress.		
	regard to work. (9) Personal accidents. (10) Accidents among family or close friends. (11) Arguments or problems with family or close social contacts. (12) Other events which were noteworthy.		
Longino, C.F., Lipman, A. (1980)	488 noninstitutionalized residents of retirement communities	—	(1) Married have more primary relations than unmarried. (2) Unmarried have more secondary relationships. (3) Among the unmarried, women received more emotional, social and instrumental support from family members. (4) Selectivity of the sample (retirement communities) may have some effect on findings.
		Primary and secondary relationships.	
Lopata, H.Z. (1978)	1169 Chicago area widows: three-quarters were widowed before reaching age 65.	—	(1) Children and parents in the case of younger widows were frequent contributors to the support system. (2) Extended kin (cousins, siblings, nephews, nieces even grandchildren contributed infrequently). (3) Male kin do not play a significant role in the emotional support system. (4) Few widows give to or receive from kin service support.
		Social, emotional, economic, and service support systems	

Author(s) (date)	Sample or Study Design	Measure of Life Change Events	Measure of Social Support	Measure of Health	Findings
Lowenthal, M.F., Haven, C. (1968)	N = 280 aged 60+	Social losses in role and interaction	Availability of a confidante	(1) Self reported well-being (2) professional appraisal of mental health.	The presence of an intimate relationship serves as a buffer against such decrements as loss of role or reduction of social interaction. Age-linked loss of widowhood and retirement are also ameliorated by the presence of a confidante but the assault of physical illness is not.
Maddison, D., Viola, A. (1968)	N = 357 Female Boston = 132 Sydney = 243 Control N = 199 Boston = 98 Sydney = 101 Widows of men who died between age 45–60 Mailed Questionnaire Retrospective matched control	Widowhood	—	Self-assessed health	(1) It was hypothesized that there is an association between health deterioration and bereavement—that rate of illness will increase following death of spouse. (2) Widows had a higher rate of health complaints during the year following bereavement than a matched nonbereaved population during a similar period.
Martin, J., Doran, A.	700 employees who experienced compulsory retirement in England Longitudinal study	Retirement	—	Self-reported illness	(1) Increasing incidence of illness requiring medical treatment in 2 years before retirement. (2) Illness rates dropped after retirement event but increased again four to six years after retirement.

Minkler, M. (1981)	Literature review	Retirement	—	Variety of measures subjective and objective measures of health.	(1) Study reviews literature and concludes that the effect of retirement on health and use of services has not been clearly determined. (2) Methodological difficulties include (a) viewing retirement as a static event rather than a process, (b) confounding retirement with declines in health status and income and (3) failure to consider the timing of event in life cycle.
Myers, J.K., Lindenthal, J.J., Pepper, M.P. (1975)	$N = 720$ (18 +). Same as 1972 study. New Haven sample Longitudinal study	List developed by Myers et al. based on Antonovsky and Katz (1967); Holmes and Rahe and additional items.	—	Mental Health Index based on MacMillan (1957) and Gurin et al., (1960)	(1) It was hypothesized that the level of social integration is associated with the relationship between life events and psychiatric symptomatology and changes in that relationship over two years. (2) Persons who report many life events and few symptoms are of higher social class position, married, satisfied with their instrumental roles, and have less frequently visited MDs or been hospitalized for a physical illness. People who have ready and meaningful access to others, feel integrated into the system, and are satisfied with their roles seem better able to cope with the impact of life events.

Author(s) (date)	Sample or Study Design	Measure of Life Change Events	Measure of Social Support	Measure of Health	Findings
Murdock, S.H., Schwartz, D.F. (1978)	$N = 160$ Elderly native Americans living on a reservation.	—	Living Arrangement: (1) alone, (2) married, (3) with extended family (children)	Awareness of available services (social and health) and use of services	Levels of perceived service needs, awareness of service agencies, and use of agency services are higher for those living in extended family settings.
Nelson, L., Winter, M. (1975)	$N = 75$ Age 62+ Noninstitutionalized	—	—	—	(1) Consideration of moving was moderately associated with the occurrence of major life disruptions and strongly associated with low-level personal independence and reduced housing and neighborhood satisfaction.
Niemi, T. (1979)	$N = 1176$ Men born in 1899. Retired on old-age pension in 1964 in Finland.	Retirement	Spouse as the source of social support	Subjects had fairly good health at the time of retirement. Comparison was made between groups on mortality and cause of death.	(1) This study hypothesized that the fewer objects there are available to the individual upon retirement, the greater is the increase in mortality after retirement. (2) No statistically significant differences in mortality between groups on the basis of marital status, could be found, although the results tended to favor the hypothesis. (3) The number of accidents and suicides exceeded the expected values but were distributed fairly evenly between the different groups. Contrary to the

Niemi, T. (1979)	$N = 939$ married men retired on old age pension in Finland. 174 had lost their spouse after retirement.	Retirement and the following of spouse's death.	(1) Mortality rate of the retired husband following the spouse's death. (2) Causes of death.	hypothesis, most of the suicides had occurred in the married group. (1) The study failed to show that the death of a wife had an effect on the retired husband that could be measured by increased mortality in the long term. (2) but, during the first six months following spouse's death, more than the expected number of retired husbands died. (3) the number of those dying either of circulatory diseases or tumors within 6 months of the spouse's death did exceed the expected values.
Nimei, T. (1980)	$N = 1176$ Men retired on old age pension in Finland.	Retirement due to old age alone.	—	Retirement did not result in the increase of mortality or any long-term or short-term effects on mortality.
Nuckolls, K.B., et al. (1972)	$N = 170$ Army wives giving birth at military hospital.	Scored for self-reported life change.	Called psychosocial assets.	Complications of pregnancy. 91 percent of women with high life change and low social support experienced complications compared with 33 percent who had high life change and high social support.

Author(s) (date)	Sample or Study Design	Measure of Life Change Events	Measure of Social Support	Measure of Health	Findings
Palmore, E., et al. (1979)	N = 375 Age 45-70 white	5 events (1) respondent's retirement (2) spouses retirement (3) widowhood (4) departure of last child from home (5) major medical event	Called social resources (1) income (2) education (3) density and availability of network	(1) self-rated (2) weight and blood pressure (3) MD visits	Major medical events were the events most likely to be followed by statistically significant change toward poor health. The two retirement events were followed by more significant declines in health than departure of last child and widowhood. In all cases when events were followed by significant declines in health they tended to be ameliorated by high resources. No statistically significant differences for age and sex.
Penrose, R.J.J. (1972)	N = 44 Aged 20-65 admitted to hospital with confirmed diagnosis of subarachnoid hemmorhage (SAH) Retrospect	Brown-Birley Schedule	—	Incidence of SAH	(1) It was hypothesized that there is an increase in life events immediately prior to SAH. (2) The group with SAH and no aneurysms had significantly more emotional disturbance immediately before onset.
Pesznecker, B.L., McNeil, J. (1975)	N = 536 98 percent white 2 percent nonwhite Females = 300 Males = 236 Systematic selection of persons listed in a commercial householder directory (aged 18-72)	SRE	Called social asset degree of interpersonal security in past and present life included information on marital status, living arrangement, number of children and close friends.	Self-reported "major change in health"	Magnitude of life events was the most important variable in explaining variance in health, but the data did not support the hypothesized tempering effect of social assets.

Pilisuk, M Froland, C (1978)	Literature review	Article classified several measures of support	(1) Two basic forms of social support: family and kinship ties an individual's broader social network, (2) Dimensions of the social network include the source—the social context of the link; frequency—number of times contact takes place; (3) duration—how long the link has been established; (4) symmetry—balance of exchange across the link; (5) intensity—degree of commitment in a link; (6) intimacy—degree of closeness in a link; (7) multiplexity—number of role relations
Pratt, L. (1972)	$N = 510$ 273 families 237 additional wives	— Characteristics of marital relationship (1) distribution of conjugal power, (2) sex role difference; (3) companionship	Level of health and health behavior (1) total symptoms (2) lifetime health status (3) present health status (4) health-care practice (5) use of preventive services (6) total use of services health knowledge (1) Conjugal power—husbands with equality in conjugal power scored significantly higher in use of health services and knowledge. For wives, this type of marriage was related to health indices 2–6. (2) Sex-role differentiation—low role differentiation was associated high level health and health behavior. (3) Companionship—the higher the level of husband-wife companionship, the higher the level of health practices, use of professional health services, and health knowledge.

Author(s) (date)	Sample or Study Design	Measure of Life Change Events	Measure of Social Support	Measure of Health	Findings
Rahe, R.H., Mahan, J.L., Arthur, R.J. (1970)	N = 2463 males Naval and Marine personnel on three naval cruisers Quasiprospective	SRE	—	New illness events using health records	(1) What kind of illness prediction LCU totals allow? Would there be a linear relationship between LCU magnitude and near-future illness? (2) There was found a low-order positive relationship between life change intensity and number of reported illnesses. A linear relationship was seen between the subjects' recent life-change intensities and illness rates.
Rahe, R.H., Arthur, R.J. (1968)	N = 3265 Naval personnel Retrospective	Military version of SRE	—	Self-reported illness episodes	(1) How many of the life changes occurring around the time of an illness are really a result rather than a cause of the illness episode. (2) Life change data seen prior to illness experience confirmed previous work done on life stress buildup prior to illness onset. Life change data seen following illness experience was a reversed and nearly symmetrical picture of events prior to illness. This suggests validity to the argument that life change has a resultant rather than causal relationship to illness.

Reference	Sample/Design		Measure		Outcome	Results
Rahe, R.H., McKean, J.D., Arthur, R.J. (1967)	$N = 50$ male Navy and Marine personnel discharged because of psychiatric illness Longitudinal analysis	—	SRE occurrence of events obtained from record	—	Medical records incidence of illness using Hinkles illness secuity scale.	(1) There is a positive association between life-changes and illness. (2) A cluster year of life—hanges were seen to occur immediately prior to an illness or clustering of illnesses. More severe illnesses were preceded by cluster-years of higher life-change magnitude than years prior to minor illnesses.
Rahe, R.H., Meyer, M., Smith, M., Kjaer, G., Holmes, T.H., (1964)	7 patient samples representing 5 medical entities a control random selection and matching for controls systemic selection.	—	SRE	—	Presence of specific disease or medical condition	(1) It was hypothesized that change in social status achieve the significance of etiological parameters and become a necessary, but not sufficient cause of disease and help explain the specificity of time of onset. (2) The mounting frequency of changes in social status found during the 2 years preceding disease onset was termed the psychological life crisis. It was postulated that the life crisis represents a necessary but not sufficient precipitation of major health changes.
Ries, W., Lutkins, S. (1967)	—	—	—	—	—	Widowed men experience poorer mental health.

Author(s) (date)	Sample or Study Design	Measure of Life Change Events	Measure of Social Support	Measure of Health	Findings
Rubin, R.T., Gunderson, E.K.E., Arthur, R.J. (1971)	N = 1005 males enlisted Naval personnel on battle ship Quasiprospective	SRE modified	—	Number of illness events using health records	(1) It was hypothesized that onset of illness is related to increased life change. (2) Subjects with higher total life change scores based on standard scoring system tended to have greater numbers of illnesses, but this scoring system was of little predictive use. Scoring based on a stepwise multiple regression analysis did significantly discriminate future illness.
Ruch, L.O., Holmes, T.H., (1970)	Adults 21 to 60 years N = 394 Adolescents Mean age 18 N = 211	List from Holmes and Rahe's Social Readjustment Rating Scale (43 events)	—	—	When the adolescent sample was compared to the adult sample, there was a general value consensus about the seriousness of life events. The analysis also revealed that the direct (magnitude estimation) and indirect (paired comparisons) scaling methods produced similar scales of life events when applied to the same population.
Shanas, E. (1979)	1975 national probability sample. Study of noninstitutionalized persons 65 years and over.	—	(1) Immediate family (spouse and children). (2) Extended family, siblings and other relatives.	—	(1) Main source of help for bedfast person was from husband or wife; children are the next source of help. (2) The extended family is the major tie of the elderly to the community.

| Skinner, H., Lei, H. (1980) | 353 alcohol and drug abuse patients; mean age 33.7 years. | Schedule of Recent Events (Holmes and Rahe) | — | — | (1) Study identified six distinct clusters of events (a) personal and social activities, (b) work changes, (c) marital problems, (d) residence changes, (e) family issues, (f) school changes. (2) Significant correlations were found between the above six clusters and the Cornell Medical Index and measures of psychopathology. (3) Physical symptoms were related to the personal change factor (4) Psychopathology and alcohol and drug abuse were related to all six scales. |
| Somers, A.R. (1979) | Literature review | — | — | — | From the review of literature it was concluded that (1) among both men and women at every age, married persons, on the average, live longer than the single, widowed or divorced. (2) Married persons generally make less use of health care services. (3) The influence of marital status toward physical or mental illness is less strong today than before due to (1) changing perceptions of health, illness and need for health care; (2) declining role of the family in health and concurrent rise in public and community supports. |

Author(s) (date)	Sample or Study Design	Measure of Life Change Events	Measure of Social Support	Measure of Health	Findings
Slesinger, D. (1976)	$N = 1174$ Black females with children ages 6 months through 11 years.	—	Primary group relationship (1) family setting (2) Visitation with and relatives Secondary group relationships (1) T.V. viewing (2) Clubs and organizations (3) Church attendance	Use of preventive medical services.	Women living in traditional family settings (with husband and children) have the highest preventive medical score. Mothers who rarely visit friends and/or relatives have a lower score on the preventive medical behavior index. Mothers who rarely watch T.V. who do not belong to clubs or organizations, and who rarely or never attend church are all below the mean in their preventive medical behavior, and are significantly different from those who do participate in these activities.
Smith, R.T. (1979)	$N = 770$ disability applicants aged 20–64	—	Called informal social networks which included family and peers (not specific)	Level of disability	Evidence suggests informal social networks play an important role in the rehabilitation of the disabled, and lay-initiative may constitute another effective resource in the process of recovery.
Thoits, P. (1980)	18–50 years. low income Single–$9,000 Married–$11,000	Negative life events "culturally defined" Prospective Study.	—	Psychopathological distress	(1) Undesirable events increase psychophysiological distress, (2) Undesirable events more related to physiological than psychological symptoms, (3) When effects of health-related problems controlled, other undesirable events have no effects on psychophysiological distress.

Walker, K., et al. (1977)	Literature review	—	Network is considered in terms of size, strength of ties, density, homogeneity of membership, dispersion of membership	—	(1) Literature suggest that a dense, homogeneous network with strong ties and low dispersion most likely to meet needs of widows in early stages of bereavement. (2) During later stages of bereavement, there is less need for emotional support and empathy and more need for information and new social contacts to aid in reorganization of life.
Wan, T.T.H., Weissert, W (forthcoming)	1,871 patients involved in day care or homemaker experiment.	—	Scale of 6 items which indicated presence of absence of social contacts with (1) spouse, (2) children, (3) siblings, (4) grandchildren, (5) other relatives, (6) friends.	(1) ADL functioning, (2) MSQ (3) Institutionalization.	(1) Social-support networks had a positive effect on patient status. (2) Availability of siblings, other relatives and friends associated with high levels of physical and mental functioning. (3) Living with others and having children was inversely related to the likelihood of institutionalization.
Wyler, A.R., Masuda, M. Holmes, T.H. (1971)	$N = 232$ hospitalized $M = 131$ $F = 101$ Aged 18–65 + Self-administered questionnaire. Cross-sectional retrospective	SRE with SRRS	—	SIRS Seriousness of Illness. Rating Scale	(1) It was hypothesized that there is a positive relationship between the amount of life change prior to the onset of illness and the seriousness of that illness. (2) A significant positive relationship of life events to illness magnitude was found. When diseases were separated into acute and chronic, only chronic showed a highly significant positive correlation.

Bibliography

Atchley, R., "Dimensions of Widowhood in Later Life," *The Gerontologist* 15 (1975):176–178.

Berardo, F., "Survivorship and Social Isolation: The Case of the Aged Widower," *The Family Coordinator* 19 (1970):11–25.

Blazer, D., "Life Events, Mental Health Functioning and the Use of Health Care Services by the Elderly," *American Journal of Public Health* 70 (1980):1174–1179.

Burch, J., "The Bereavement in Relation to Suicide," *Journal of Psychosomatic Research* 16 (1972):361–366.

Casscells, W., et al., "Retirement and Coronary Mortality," *The Lancet* (June 14, 1980), pp. 1288–1289.

Cobb, S., "Social Support as a Moderator of Life Stress," *Psychosomatic Medicine* 38 (1976):300–312.

Cohen, S.I., and J. Hajioff, "Life Events and the Onset of Acute Closed-Angle Glaucoma," *Journal of Psychosomatic Research* 16 (1972): 335–341.

Crisp, A.H., and R.G. Priest, "Psychoneurotic Status During the Year Following Bereavement," *Journal of Psychosomatic Research* 16 (1972): 351–355.

Croog, S.H., et al., "Help Patterns: The Roles of Kin Network, Non-Family Resources, and Institutions," *Journal of Marriage and the Family* 2 (1972):32–41.

Dean, A., et al., "Relating Types of Social Support to Depression in the Life Course," paper presented at the annual meetings of the American Sociological Association, New York, August 1980.

DeArajuo, G., et al. "Life Change, Coping Ability and Chronic Intrinsic Asthma," *Journal of Psychosomatic Research* 17 (1973):359–363.

Eaton, W.W., "Life Events, Social Supports, and Psychiatric Symptoms," *Journal of Health and Social Behavior* 19 (1978):230–234.

Eckenrode, J., and S. Gore, "Stressful Events and Social Supports: The Significance of Context," in B.H. Gottlieb, ed., *Social Networks and Social Support in Community Mental Health* (Beverly Hills, Calif.: Sage Publications, 1981).

Elwell, F., and A.D. Maltbie-Crannell, "The Impact of Role Loss Upon Coping Resources and Life Satisfaction of the Elderly," *Journal of Gerontology* 36 (1981):223–232.

Fenwich, R., and C.M. Barresi, "Health Consequences of Marital-Status Change Among the Elderly," *Journal of Health and Social Behavior* 22 (1981):106–116.

Fillenbaum, G.G., "Social Context and Self-Assessments of Health Among the Elderly," *Journal of Health and Social Behavior* 14 (1979): 167–175.

Finlayson, A., "Social Networks as Coping Resources," *Social Science and Medicine* 10 (1976):47–103.

Foner, A., and S. Schwab, *Aging and Retirement* (Monterey, Calif.: Brooks/Cole Publishing Co., 1980).

Fuller, S.S., and S.B. Larson, "Life Events, Emotional Support, and Health of Older People," *Research in Nursing and Health* 3 (1980): 81–89.

Gelein, J.L., "The Aged American Female: Relationships Between Social Support and Health," *Journal of Gerontological Nursing* 6 (1980): 69–73.

George, L.K., and G.L. Maddox, "Subjective Adaptation to Loss of the Work Role: A Longitudinal Study," *Journal of Gerontology* 32 (1977): 456–462.

Goldberg, E.L., and G.W. Comstock, "Epidemiology of Life Events: Frequency in General Populations," *American Journal of Epidemiology* 111 (1980):736–752.

Guttman, D., "Life Events and Decision Making by Older Adults," *The Gerontologist* 18 (1978):5.

Heyman, D.K., and D.T. Gianturco, "Long-Term Adaptation by the Elderly to Bereavement," *Journal of Gerontology* 28 (1973):359–362.

Holtzman, J.M., et al., "Health and Early Retirement Decisions," *Journal of the American Geriatrics Society* 28 (1980):23–28.

Horwitz, A., "Family, Kin, and Friend Networks in Psychiatric Help-Seeking," *Social Science and Medicine* 12 (1978):297–304.

Justice, B., "Life Events, Level of Distress, and Social Supports in Graduate Student Population," paper presented at the Annual Meeting of the American Public Health Association in Detroit, Mich., 1980.

Kaplan, B.H., et al., "Social Support and Health," *Medical Care* 15 (1977):47–58.

Kimmel, D.C., K.S. Price, and J.W. Walker, "Retirement Choice and Retirement Satisfaction," *Journal of Gerontology* 33 (1978):575–585.

Langlie, J.K., "Social Networks, Health Beliefs and Preventive Health Behavior," *Journal of Health and Social Behavior* 18 (1977):244–260.

Lin, N., et al., "Social Support, Stressful Life Events, and Illness: A Model and an Empirical Test," *Journal of Health and Social Behavior* 20 (1979):108–119.

Linn, M.W., et al., "Symptoms of Depression and Recent Life Events in the Community Elderly," *Journal of Clinical Psychology* 36 (1980): 675–682.

Longino, D.F., and A. Lipman, "Married and Spouseless Men and Women in Planned Retirement Communities: Support Network Differentials," paper presented at the thirty-second Annual Meeting of the Gerontological Society, Washington, D.C., 1979.

Lopata, H.Z., "Contributions of Extended Families to the Social Support

Systems of Metropolitan Area Widows: Limitations of the Modified Kin Network," *Journal of Marriage and the Family* 40 (1979):358–364.

Lowenthal, M.F., and C. Haven, "Interaction and Adaptation: Intimacy as a Critical Valuable," *American Sociological Review* 33 (1968): 20–30.

Maddison, D., and A. Violà., "The Health of Widows in the Year Following Bereavement," *Journal of Psychosomatic Research* 12 (1968): 297–306.

Martin, J., and A. Doran, "Evidence Concerning the Relationship Between Health and Retirement," *Sociological Review* 14 (1966):329.

Minkler, M., "Research on the Health Effects of Retirement: An Uncertain Legacy," *Journal of Health and Social Behavior* 22 (1981):117–130.

Murdock, S.H., and D.F. Schwartz, "Family Structure and the Use of Agency Services: An Examination of Patterns Among Elderly Native Americans," *The Gerontologist* 18 (1978):475–481.

Myers, J.K., et al., "Life Events, Social Integration, and Psychiatric Symptomology," *Journal of Health and Social Behavior* 16 (1975):421–427.

Nelson, L., and Winter, M., "Life Disruption, Independence, Satisfaction and Consideration of Moving," *The Gerontologist* 15 (1978):160–164.

Niemi, T., "The Mortality of Male Old-Age Pensioners Following Spouses' Death," *Scandanavian Journal of Social Medicine* 7 (1979):115–117.

Niemi, T., "Effect of Loneliness on Mortality After Retirement," *Scandanavian Journal of Social Medicine* 7 (1979):63–65.

Niemi, T., "Retirement and Mortality," *Scandanavian Journal of Social Medicine* 8 (1980):39–41.

Nuckolls, K.B., et al., "Psychosocial Assets, Life Crisis and the Prognosis of Pregnancy," *American Journal of Epidemiology* 95 (1972):431–441.

Palmore, E., et al., "Stress and Adaptation in Later Life," *Journal of Gerontology* 34 (1979):841–851.

Penrose, R.J.J., "Life Events Before Subarachnois Hemorrhage," *Journal of Psychosomatic Research* 16 (1972):329–333.

Pesznecker, B.C., and J. McNeil, "Relationship Among Health Habits, Social Assets, Psychologic Well-Being, Life Change, and Alterations in Health Status," *Nursing Research* 24 (1975):442–447.

Pilisuk, M., and C. Froland, "Kinship, Social Networks, Social Support and Health," *Social Science and Medicine* 12 (1978):273–280.

Pratt, J., "Conjugal Organization and Health," *Journal of Marriage and the Family* 34 (1972):85–94.

Rahe, R.H., et al., "Social Stress and Illness Onset," *Journal of Psychosomatic Research* 8 (1964):35–44.

Rahe, R.H., J.D. McKean, R.J. Arthur, "A Longitudinal Study of Life-Change and Illness Patterns," *Journal of Psychosomatic Research* 10 (1966):355–366.

Rahe, R.H., and R.J. Arthur, "Life Change Patterns Surrounding Illness Experience," *Journal of Psychosomatic Research* 11 (1968):341-345.

Rahe, R.H., J. Mahan, and R.J. Arthur, "Prediction of Near-Future Health Changes from Subjects Preceding Life Changes," *Journal of Psychosomatic Research* 14 (1970):401-406.

Rees, W., and S. Lutkins, "The Mortality of Bereavement," *British Medical Journal,* January 1967.

Ruch, L.O., and T.H. Holmes, "Scaling of Life Change: Comparison of Direct and Indirect Methods," *Journal of Psychosomatic Research* 15 (1970):221-227.

Shanas, E., "The Family as a Social Support System in Old Age," *The Gerontologist* 19 (1979):169-174.

Skinner, H., and H. Lei, "The Multidimensional Assessment of Stressful Life Events," *Journal of Nervous and Mental Disorders* 247 (1980): 535-541.

Slesinger, D.P., "The Utilization of Preventive Medical Services by Urban Black Mothers," in David Mechanic, ed., *The Growth of Bureaucratic Medicine* (New York: John Wiley and Sons, 1976).

Smith, R.T., "Rehabilitation of the Disabled: The Role of Social Networks in the Recovery Process," *International Rehabilitative Medicine* 1 (1979):63-72.

Somers, A.R., "Marital Status, Health and Use of Health Services," *Journal of the American Medical Association* 241 (1979):1818-1822.

Thoits, P.A., "Undesirable Life Events and Psychophysiological Distress: A Problem of Operational Confounding," *American Sociological Review* 46 (1981):97-109.

Walker, K.N., et al., "Social Support Networks and the Crisis of Bereavement," *Social Science and Medicine* 11 (1977):35-41.

Wan, T.T.H., and W. Weissert, "Social Support Networks, Patient Status, and Institutionalization," *Research on Aging* 3, no. 2 (1981):240-256.

Wyler, A., M. Masuda, and T. Holmes, "Magnitude of Life Events and Seriousness of Illness," *Journal of Psychosomatic Medicine* 33 (1971): 115-122.

Index

About the Author

Thomas T.H. Wan is professor of health administration at the Medical College of Virginia, Virginia Commonwealth University. He is a medical sociologist who has taught at the University of Maryland Baltimore County and at Cornell University. Dr. Wan did his undergraduate work at Tunghai University in Taiwan and received the M.A. (1968) and the Ph.D. (1970) in sociology from the University of Georgia. He also received the M.H.S. (1971) from The Johns Hopkins University School of Hygiene and Public Health, where he was the National Institutes of Health postdoctoral Fellow.

Dr. Wan belongs to many professional societies; is a Fellow of the Gerontological Society of America; and serves on the Governing Council of the American Public Health Association. He has also served as a consultant to various health agencies. His current research in gerontology focuses on the determinants and consequences of institutionalization, evaluation of long-term-care programs, and gerontological health. As a health-services researcher, he has published numerous articles and books in the health-care field.